COLOR ATLAS OF
VETERINARY
HISTOLOGY
Second Edition

COLOR ATLAS OF
VETERINARY HISTOLOGY
Second Edition

William J. Bacha, Jr., PhD

Professor Emeritus
Department of Biology
Rutgers University
Camden College of Arts and Sciences
Camden, New Jersey

Linda M. Bacha, MS, VMD

Assistant Professor of Biology
Department of Biology
Camden County College
Blackwood, New Jersey

LIPPINCOTT WILLIAMS & WILKINS
A **Wolters Kluwer** Company

Philadelphia • Baltimore • New York • London
Buenos Aires • Hong Kong • Sydney • Tokyo

Editor: Donna Balado
Managing Editor: Dana Battaglia
Marketing Manager: Anne Smith
Production Editor: Jennifer D. Weir

351 West Camden Street
Baltimore, Maryland 21201-2436

530 Walnut Street
Philadelphia, Pennsylvania 19106-3621

Printed in the United States of America

First Edition, 1990

Library of Congress Cataloging-in-Publication Data

Bacha, William J.
   Color atlas of veterinary histology / William J. Bacha, Jr., Linda M. Bacha.—2nd ed.
      p. cm.
   Includes bibliographical references (p.).
   ISBN 0-683-30618-9
   1. Veterinary histology—Atlases.   I. Bacha, Linda M.   II. Title.

SF757.3.B33 2000
636.089'1018—dc21   99-046388

To purchase additional copies of this book, call our customer service department at (800) **638-3030** or fax orders to (301) **824-7390**. International customers should call (301) **714-2324**.

                                        03   04
                        4   5   6   7   8   9   10

THIS BOOK IS DEDICATED TO
JESSIE & TRISTAN

PREFACE
TO THE SECOND EDITION

We wish to thank those who have used the first edition for their suggestions. We believe the incorporation of many of these recommendations will make this edition even more helpful to the user.

To this end, we have updated the material for the second edition by scanning all of the original kodachromes and relabeling the art. We have added thirteen new photographs and have enlarged over one hundred others. Four of the original black and white line drawings have also been redrawn. Also, a glossary of nearly 750 words has been added.

The style, format, and purpose of this edition remain essentially unchanged from the first edition. We continue to view the atlas as a useful, benchside reference for those interested in understanding and interpreting histologic and cytologic preparations.

PREFACE
TO THE FIRST EDITION

Although we have written this atlas primarily to fulfill a need of the student of veterinary medicine, we believe that clinicians, private practitioners, and researchers will find it a useful reference for normal tissues and organs. Currently, students rely heavily, if not exclusively, on atlases of human histology for guidance in the laboratory. There are, of course, similarities between organs and tissues of domestic animals and those of humans. There are also differences, however, and these are rarely encountered in atlases dealing specifically with human histology.

Our aim has been to compare the histologic structure of organs in a variety of domestic animals. We have used representative examples in instances where tissues and organs from different animals share a common structure. Wherever differences exist, we have tried to provide examples that are characteristic of a particular group of animals. Our selection of animals includes the dog, cat, horse, cow, sheep, goat, pig, and chicken because they are most frequently referenced in veterinary school curricula.

All photomicrographs and drawings are original. Some drawings were done freehand, while others were made with the aid of a camera lucida. Light microscopy and colored photomicrographs have been used exclusively. We have chosen color rather than black and white because of its correspondence to stained preparations. With the exception of the few histologic preparations loaned to us by generous donors or purchased from a dealer, slides were prepared by the authors. Fresh organ samples were obtained from a slaughterhouse or from animals that were euthanized for various reasons. With the exception of smear preparations (blood, bone marrow, and vaginal), mesenteric spreads, ground bone, and a single plastic section, slides were prepared using the paraffin method. All slides were stained with hematoxylin and eosin unless otherwise noted. Magnifications of photomicrographs are total magnifications (enlargement of photograph × objective × projector lens). Throughout the atlas, hollow structures, for example, blood vessels, kidney tubules, and alveoli, are usually identified by labeling the lumen of the structure.

ACKNOWLEDGMENTS
FROM THE FIRST EDITION

Help is often just around the corner. Dr. Henry Stempen, whose office was down the hall from ours at Rutgers University in Camden, New Jersey, stopped by one day and volunteered his artistic talents. We'd like to thank him for his excellent pen and ink drawings of various animal parts, which are somewhat removed from the fungi he usually draws. Our gratitude also to Ms. Kathleen Carr for her secretarial services. Special thanks are extended to Dr. Edward Zambraski, Ms. Kathleen O'Hagan, and Ms. Gail Thomas of Cook College, Rutgers University, for making fresh porcine material available to us; and to Dr. Barry Jesse and Dr. James Harner for supplying us with sheep parts.

Without the unqualified use of the facilities and equipment of the Biology Department of Rutgers, our tissue processing and photomicrography could not have been accomplished. Our special thanks to the Department for this courtesy.

This book would never have had a beginning were it not for the generosity of Dr. Leon Weiss, Department of Animal Biology, University of Pennsylvania School of Veterinary Medicine, who invited us to teach in the veterinary histology laboratory and kindly allowed us access to the slide collection and facilities of the Department. We would also like to express appreciation to the following individuals from the University of Pennsylvania School of Veterinary Medicine: Mr. Richard Aucamp and Mrs. Kathy Aucamp, who provided us with specimens, slides, advice, and assistance in a variety of other ways; Dr. mark Haskins for kindly making available fresh canine and feline material; Dr. John Fyfe and Dr. Vicki Meyers-Wallen for supplying us with canine vaginal smears; Dr. and Mrs. Loren Evans and Dr. David McDevitt for lending us reference material; Dr. Peter Hand and Ms. Graziella Mann for providing material on the nervous system; and Dr. Helen Acland, Dr. Linda Bachin, Mr. James Bruce, Dr. Sherrill Davison, Ms. Dawn Dowling, Dr. Robert Dyer, Dr. Robert Eckroade, Dr. George Farnbach, Dr. David Freeman, Dr. Wendy Freeman, Dr. Alan Kelly, Mr. Joseph McGrane, and Dr. Mary Sommer for thcir time and consideration in helping us to obtain tissue specimens.

We are grateful to Dr. Carol Jacobson and the Department of Anatomy of the Iowa State University College of Veterinary Medicine for providing valuable slide preparations and text material.

Our gratitude is also extended to Hill's Pet Products, Topeka, Kansas, and Pitman-Moore, Inc., Washington Crossing, New Jersey, for their generous financial assistance.

Many thanks also to: Dr. Caroline Czarnecki of the University of Minnesota, College of Veterinary Medicine, for providing copies of her informative laboratory guide; Dr. Deborah Ganster, Dr. James Lawhead, Dr. Virginia Pierce, Dr. Maria Salvaggio, Dr. Barbara Strock, and Dr. Cindi Ward for assisting us in obtaining tissue samples; Mr. Jeff Bringhurst, Bringhurst Brothers, Tansboro, New Jersey, for allowing us access to fresh large animal material; the Longenecker Hatchery, Elizabethtown, Pennsylvania, for providing chicken specimens; Ms. Susan Ulrich, Cornell University Press, for lending us a difficult-to-obtain reference; the helpful people at Optical Apparatus Company Inc., Ardmore, Pennsylvania, for supplies and for assistance with equipment for the microscope; and to Mr. Charles Behl and Mr. James Durso of Webb and Company Inc., Cherry Hill, New Jersey, for their courteous service and helpful advice.

We are indebted to Mr. William J. Bacha, Sr., for building a super light box for us, and to Mr. Thomas H. Wood, Jr., for providing black and white prints of our photomicrographs, which saved us countless hours of drudgery in the darkroom. Thanks to Barbara Frasco, Esq., for her helpful advice. Our hats are off also to Snuff, Chew, Chapter Seat, Angel, Clyde, and all the other animals for their participation.

We also wish to extend our gratitude to all at Lippincott Williams & Wilkins whose efforts helped bring this second edition into being. We are especially grateful to Carroll C. Cann and Jennifer D. Weir for their professional advice, courtesy, and assistance.

William J. Bacha, Jr
Linda M. Bacha

CONTENTS

1

GENERAL PRINCIPLES OF HISTOLOGY

PREPARATION OF HISTOLOGIC SECTIONS

A histologic section is a thin slice of tissue varying, usually, from 0.5 to 10 or more micrometers (μm) thick. In preparing such a section, a piece of tissue is either infiltrated with a supporting medium or frozen and is then cut with an instrument called a microtome. Sections obtained from tissue infiltrated with plastic can be as thin as 0.5 μm and show superior detail. Excellent preparations as thin as 2 or 3 μm can also be made from tissue infiltrated with paraffin-based embedding media. Sections are affixed to microscope slides and colored with one or more stains to increase the visibility of various cellular and intercellular components.

Schematically, Figure 1.1 outlines various steps involved in producing a stained histologic slide using the paraffin procedure. After being removed from an animal, a tissue or organ is cut into pieces. These pieces are placed into a fixative such as buffered formalin or Bouin's, which, ideally, preserves normal morphology and facilitates further processing. After fixation, the specimen is dehydrated by transferring it through a series of alcohols of increasing concentrations to 100% alcohol. Next, it is placed into a substance such as xylene, or xylene substitute, which is miscible with both 100% alcohol and paraffin. This intermediate step (called clearing) is essential before infiltrating the dehydrated tissue with paraffin because alcohol and paraffin do not mix. During infiltration, melted paraffin completely replaces the xylene. This procedure is done in an oven at a temperature just above the melting point of the paraffin. When infiltration is complete, the specimen is transferred to an embedding mold of fresh paraffin, which is allowed to harden. Then the mold is removed and excess paraffin is trimmed away.

The block of paraffin is then secured to the microtome and oriented appropriately with respect to the knife. With each revolution of the microtome handle, the specimen moves through the blade and a section of the desired thickness is produced. Each successive section adheres to the preceding one, forming a continuous ribbon. Subsequently, one or more sections are carefully separated from the ribbon and transferred to the surface of

1

1. Removing Organ Sample

2. Cutting Small Pieces

3. Preparing Specimens for Sectioning

Fix

Dehydrate

Clear

Embed

Mold with Specimen in Melted Paraffin

Paraffin Block Removed from Mold

Trimmed Block

4. Sectioning with Microtome

HSTEMPEN

5. Straightening Sections on Waterbath

6. Transferring Sections to Slide

7. Drying on Warmer

8. Staining

9. Coverslipping

Figure 1.1. The various steps involved in producing a histologic slide using the paraffin method.

warm water in a waterbath. This softens the paraffin and flattens the section, eliminating wrinkles. The flattened section is floated onto a slide, which is then placed on a warming table. As the preparation dries, the section adheres to the surface of the slide.

Next, the paraffin is removed with xylene or another appropriate solvent and the specimen is rehydrated. It is then stained, dehydrated, cleared (made transparent) with xylene, covered with a resinous mounting medium, and topped with a cover-slip.

Various stains are available to the histologist. Hematoxylin and eosin (H&E) is a frequently used combination of stains. Hematoxylin imparts a purple color to substances, but must be linked to a metallic salt called a mordant before it can function effectively. This combination, called a lake, carries a positive charge and behaves as a basic (cationic) stain. The lake combines electrostatically with negatively charged radicals such as phosphate groups of nucleoproteins. Substances that become colored by a basic stain are said to be basophilic. Methylene blue, toluidine blue, and basic fuchsin are basic stains. Unlike hematoxylin, these stains have molecules that carry a positive charge of their own and do not require a mordant. Acidic (anionic) stains carry a negative charge and color cell or tissue components that bear positive charges. Eosin is an acid stain. It imparts an orange or red color to acidophilic substances. Other commonly used acid stains are orange G, phloxine, and aniline blue.

In addition to the widely used H&E staining procedure, numerous other stain combinations and techniques are available. Some are especially useful for identifying certain tissue elements. For example, trichrome procedures such as Mallory's and Masson's specifically stain collagenous fibers within connective tissue. Orcein and Weigert's resorcin fuchsin are stains used to color elastic fibers, providing a means of distinguishing them from other fibrous elements. Reticular fibers and nervous tissue components such as neurons, myelin, and cells of the neuroglia can be stained by procedures employing the use of silver. There are also special histochemical and immunohistochemical procedures that make possible the localization of various carbohydrates, lipids, and proteins found in tissue. Lastly, stains such as Wright's and Giemsa's (Romanovsky stains) are available for differentiating the various cells found in blood and bone marrow.

INTERPRETING SECTIONS

One must know the gross structure of an organ before a histologic section from it can be comprehended. It is also helpful to know how the section was cut, that is, whether it was a cross section (x.s.), a longitudinal section (l.s.), or an oblique slice through the organ. Was the cut made through the entire organ or only through a portion of it? Frequently, prepared slides are labeled indicating the particular orientation of the section. This is not important in an asymmetric organ such as the spleen or liver because their appearance would be unaffected by the direction of the cut. Conversely, the small intestine is radially symmetric and its appearance is affected by the direction of the cut.

The three-dimensional structure of organs and their components must also be considered when examining a histologic preparation. Cells are three-dimensional objects differing in size and shape. For example, some are long and thin, some cuboidal, and others ovoid. They may have a random or specific arrangement within an organ. How they appear depends on their shape, as well as how they were cut. Imagine how the spindle-shaped and tall columnar cells shown in Figure 1.2A would look if sectioned in various planes. Note that the nucleus may or may not be included in a particular cut through a cell.

The histologist examines multicellular structures having a wide variety of shapes. Some are hollow, some branch repeatedly, some open onto surfaces, etc. Figure 1.2, B and C, and Figure 1.3 show a variety of three-dimensional structures and how they would appear if cut at different levels. Examine these carefully. They will help you to understand situations you will encounter on actual slides.

HELPFUL HINTS

Be sure that the lenses of your microscope are clean before you begin examining slides. Use a piece of lens paper or a soft, clean cloth such as an old (but clean) linen handkerchief. If the lenses have been coated with oil or another substance, remove it using lens tissue moistened sparingly with a glass cleaner such as Windex. Slides should also be cleaned using a soft, lint-free cloth or tissue moistened with glass cleaner.

Every microscope should have a pointer in the ocular. This is usually supplied by the manufacturer, but can be made from a short piece of hair. The latter is cemented into place inside the ocular with a dab of quick-drying glue or nail polish. Without a pointer, it is not possible to accurately indicate an object in the microscope field for another observer.

Before beginning a session at the microscope, make sure that the fine-adjustment knob is near the middle of its range of rotation. If you do not, you may find that the knob is at the limit of its excursion when you are busily making observations. At that point, you must stop everything and correct it.

It is also a good habit to examine your slide with the unaided eye before placing it on the stage of your microscope. If you do so, you will gain information about the gross aspects of the specimen and be more likely to center it properly over the light source. Centering is especially important for small specimens that might otherwise be difficult to locate. Also, make sure that you put the slide on the stage with the cover glass uppermost. If the slide is upside down, you will not be able to focus on it with the high-power lenses. Do not snicker. We have seen this happen often in the teaching laboratory!

It is always a good idea to start your observations using the lowest power objective available on your microscope. This is usually the 4× lens. The field of view will be large, enabling you to locate regions of special interest more easily. When you locate something you wish to examine at a higher magnification, center the object in the

Figure 1.2. A. Slices, indicated by numbered planes, taken through two different types of cells would appear as identified by the prime numbers. Only if the plane of the cut passes through the nucleus will the latter be seen. **B and C.** Planes of section taken from different levels in four separate multicellular objects are illustrated. Note how the appearance of sections varies with the level of the cut.

Figure 1.3. The prime numbers illustrate sections resulting from transverse (**4**), oblique (**1**), and longitudinal (**2,3,5,6**) cuts made through a plate of cells bearing hollow projections *(above plate)* and invaginations *(below plate)*. Plane 3 differs from the others because it passes only through the cellular wall of a projection, and not the lumen; therefore, section 3′ appears as a plate of cells rather than a hollow structure. You should also be aware that structures may often appear unrelated to a surface or another object, when in fact they are. Compare planes 5 and 6 with sections 5′ and 6′, where continuity of the invagination with the surface is evident only in 6 and 6′. While not apparent from a single section, such continuity would be evident if an uninterrupted series of sections through the entire invagination were made and examined.

middle of the field of view. Then, when you change to a stronger lens, the object should be somewhere in the field.

Binocular microscopes often have at least one ocular that can be adjusted to accommodate your vision. It is important that you adjust this properly if you want to have a comfortable, headache-free session at the microscope. Assuming that your microscope is of the binocular type and that it has at least one adjustable ocular, you should first bring the specimen into focus with the ocular that is not adjustable by using the fine adjustment knob. When you have done this, focus the other eye using the adjustable ocular. Use of this procedure will ensure a proper focus for both eyes and prevent eye strain.

Bright, even lighting is absolutely essential to effective microscopy. The best way to achieve this is to use Köhler illumination. This can be obtained with any microscope that is equipped with both a condenser aperture diaphragm (the one in the condenser) and a field diaphragm (the one in the light source). If you have such an instrument, proceed as follows:

1. Center the light source, using the directions you received with the microscope.
2. Open both the field and aperture diaphragms fully.
3. Raise the condenser to its uppermost position.
4. Place a specimen on the stage and focus on it using the 10X objective.
5. Close the field diaphragm so that its leaves are clearly imaged in the field of view.
6. Center the image of the diaphragm by manipulating the condenser centering screws, then open the field diaphragm until its leaves disappear just beyond the edge of the field of view.
7. Remove an ocular and, while looking into the back aperture of the objective, close the aperture diaphragm completely and then open it until it is about 75% of being fully open.

You now have Köhler illumination. If you want to increase or decrease the light intensity, use the rheostat or neutral-density filters, but do not adjust the condenser aperture diaphragm or field diaphragm. If the aperture diaphragm is open to excess, the image will lack some contrast and be flooded with light. If it is closed too far, there will be a loss of resolution and increase in contrast. This increase in contrast is often confused with sharpness or high resolution; this is a common error in microscopy. All of the above adjustments (except for centering the light source) must be made each time a different objective is used.

If your microscope lacks a field diaphragm, you will not be able to obtain Köhler illumination. You can still acquire good and useful lighting, however. Place a specimen on the stage, open the aperture diaphragm fully, and adjust the light intensity with the rheostat so that it is comfortable for your eyes. Be sure that the condenser is raised to its highest position, or close to it, when you do this. Now, remove an ocular and look at the back aperture of the objective. Close the aperture diaphragm fully and then open it until it is about 75% of being fully open. This will provide proper lighting for most purposes. If you should need more or less illumination, make adjustments only with the rheostat or neutral density filter; do not use the aperture diaphragm.

To get the most from a specimen, you must avoid being a passive microscopist, that is, one who finds an object and then stares at it admiringly without making further adjustments of the focus. Get into the habit of focusing continuously with the fine adjustment as you peruse a slide, because even though a tissue section may be only a few micrometers thick, the depth of field of the higher power objectives may be less than the thickness of the specimen. Therefore, if you do not focus repeatedly as you examine a preparation, you will certainly miss seeing structural detail that might be important to your work.

You might like to return to a particular location on your slide preparation at a future time. Remembering landmarks in the vicinity of the object of interest will aid you in locating the object later. A more expedient way of relocating structures is by using verniers, which are mounted on both the X and Y axes of the mechanical stage. A vernier consists of two, parallel, graduated, sliding scales, one long and one short. The smaller scale is 9 millimeters (mm) long and is divided into 10 subdivisions (0 to 10). The larger scale is several centimeters (cm) long and is graduated in millimeters, for example, 0 to 80 or 100 to 160. To relocate an object on a slide, you must first center it in the microscope field. Once this has been done, you establish its location by reading each of the verniers (X and Y). For example, the 0 point on the small scale of the vernier on the X axis might be located somewhere between lines 42 and 43 on the larger scale (Fig. 1.4). To determine its specific location, find the line on the small scale that coincides exactly with a line on the longer scale. Then count, on the smaller scale, the number of spaces between 0 and the point of coincidence. This number is your decimal point. In the example given (Fig. 1.4), the decimal is 0.6 and you should read 42.6 as the vernier value. Do the same for the other vernier (Y) and record the numbers for both. In the future, if you want to return to the same location, simply secure the slide to the mechanical stage and move the stage controls until the verniers are adjusted to the numbers you previously recorded. These manipulations will have returned the slide to its former position, and the object you are looking for should be somewhere within the microscope field.

By knowing the approximate diameter of a red blood cell in a section, you can estimate the size of other tissue

Figure 1.4. Small and large vernier scales.

components. Therefore, it useful to know that in tissue sections prepared by the paraffin method the average size of erythrocytes for each of the following animals is as follows:

Goat   2.4 μm diameter (smallest erythrocytes of the domestic mammals)
Dog   4.9 μm diameter (largest erythrocytes of the domestic mammals)
Chicken   9.4 mm long

Each average value is based on a total of 20 to 30 cells that were measured from five different slide preparations of tissues embedded in Paraplast X-TRA (Monoject Scientific, Division of Sherwood Medical, St. Louis, MO 63103).

ARTIFACTS

Folds, knife marks, stain precipitate, spaces (where none belong), shrinkage, and air bubbles are examples of commonly occurring imperfections seen in slide preparations. They were introduced during processing and are called artifacts. Figures 1.5 through 1.9 are examples of such artifacts.

Figure 1.5.   × 62.5

Figure 1.6.   × 62.5

Figure 1.7.   × 62.5

Figure 1.8.   × 25

Figure 1.9.   × 62.5

KEY	
1. Dermis	4. Knife mark
2. Epidermis	5. Separation artifact
3. Fold	6. Stain precipitate

Figure 1.5. Stain Precipitate, Cartilage, Dog. Occasionally, solutions accumulate precipitate that may stick to the surface of tissue sections during the staining procedure.

Figure 1.6. Separation (space) Artifact, Skin, Dog. Tissues may be subjected to excessive pressures, tensions, or shrinkage during processing, resulting in separations within otherwise intact tissue.

Figure 1.7. Crackling Artifact, Thymus, Horse. Highly cellular tissues, for example, thymus, liver, pancreas, and spleen, often show numerous tiny cracks throughout. Also note that this specimen is not in sharp focus.

Figure 1.8. Knife Marks and Folds, Esophagus, Horse (Masson's). Knife marks (scratches) in the tissue section may be caused by defects in the microtome knife or by accumulations of debris on the knife edge. Folds occur when the tissue sections fail to spread properly on the surface of the slide.

Figure 1.9. Fold, Aorta, Pig. In a tissue section, folds are raised areas that frequently overlap. Note that portions of this picture are not in sharp focus.

2

EPITHELIUM

The external and internal surfaces of the body and many of its parts are covered by one or more layers of cells. These cellular coverings or linings constitute a tissue called epithelium. Epithelial cells are supported by a basement membrane that separates them from the underlying connective tissue. Cells are the principal components of the epithelium. Intercellular substance is sparse and is exemplified by the thin layer of material located between cells, which helps to hold them together. The free surface of epithelial cells may possess cilia, microvilli, or stereocilia.

Simple epithelia consist of a single layer of cells. The latter may have a **squamous** (flattened), **cuboidal** (more or less square), or **columnar** (tall and rectangular) shape when seen in profile. **Pseudostratified columnar,** a special category of simple epithelium, appears in profile to consist of several layers of cells. This is an illusion that results from nuclei being located at different levels within cells of different heights. In a simple epithelium, all the cells are in contact with the basement membrane.

Stratified epithelia contain two or more layers of cells. Only the bottom-most layer is in contact with the basement membrane. They are classified as stratified squamous, cuboidal, or columnar, depending on the shape of those cells in their outermost (surface) layer. A category called **transitional** is a special form of stratified epithelium limited to the urinary system. The shape of its cells will vary with the amount of fluid pressure applied against it.

All glands, endocrine or exocrine, are derived from an epithelium during development. Numerous examples of glands are presented in subsequent chapters.

Figure 2.1   × 250

Figure 2.2   × 250

Figure 2.3   × 250

Figure 2.4   × 250

Figure 2.5   × 125

KEY	
1. Basal cell	9. Hepatocyte
2. Basement membrane	10. Lamina propria
3. Columnar cell	11. Lymphocyte
4. Columnar cell, ciliated	12. Smooth muscle cell
5. Connective tissue	13. Squamous cell, nucleus
6. Cuboidal cell	14. Stratified squamous epithelium
7. Esophagus, lumen	15. Striated border
8. Goblet cell	

Figure 2.1. Simple Squamous Epithelium, Mesothelium, Liver, Cat. The surface of the liver is covered by a single layer of squamous cells that lie on a thin layer of connective tissue. The cytoplasm of the squamous cells is sparse and generally only the nucleus is visible.

Figure 2.2. Simple Cuboidal Epithelium, Kidney, Cow (Trichrome). The lining of these collecting tubules consists of a layer of cuboidal cells.

Figure 2.3. Simple Columnar Epithelium, Jejunum, Dog. The jejunum is lined by a simple columnar epithelium. A striated border, consisting of numerous microvilli, is evident. Goblet cells and migrating lymphocytes are present among the columnar cells.

Figure 2.4. Ciliated Pseudostratified Columnar Epithelium, Trachea, Cow. In this epithelium the nuclei are at different levels, giving the impression of stratification. All cells, however, contact the basement membrane.

Figure 2.5. Stratified Squamous Epithelium, Nonkeratinized, Esophagus, Cat. Only cells of the basal layer contact the basement membrane. The name of this epithelium is derived from the squamous cells of its outer layer.

Figure 2.6   × 250

Figure 2.10   × 125

Figure 2.7   × 250

KEY	
1. Bistratified cuboidal epithelium	4. Smooth muscle
	5. Stratified columnar epithelium
2. Dermis	6. Transitional epithelium
3. Keratinized cells	

Figure 2.6. Stratified Squamous Epithelium, Keratinized, Wattle, Pig. The wattle is covered by a keratinized stratified squamous epithelium.

Figure 2.7. Bistratified Cuboidal Epithelium, Esophagus, Dog. Ducts of glands of the esophagus are lined by a bistratified cuboidal epithelium.

Figure 2.8. Stratified Columnar Epithelium, Urethra, Goat. This portion of the urethra is lined by a stratified columnar epithelium.

Figure 2.9. Transitional Epithelium, Unstretched, Urinary Bladder, Cat. Surface cells of the transitional epithelial lining are either balloon-shaped or broadly cuboidal when not under tension.

Figure 2.10. Transitional Epithelium, Stretched, Urinary Bladder, Cat. Surface cells of this epithelium are flattened and elongated when the bladder is full.

Figure 2.8   × 250

Figure 2.9   × 125

3

CONNECTIVE TISSUE PROPER AND EMBRYONAL CONNECTIVE TISSUE

Connective tissue binds together and supports other tissues. It is a composite of various cells and fibers in an amorphous ground substance. The latter two components comprise the extracellular matrix, which typically predominates over the cellular elements.

The **ground substance,** composed largely of glycoproteins and glycosaminoglycans, forms a well-hydrated gel that fills the spaces between cells, fibers, and vessels of connective tissue. It acts as a reservoir for interstitial fluid, providing a medium through which oxygen, nutrients, and metabolic by-products diffuse to and from cells of various tissues and the vascular system.

Collagenous, reticular, and elastic fibers occur in connective tissue. **Collagenous fibers,** composed of the fibrous protein collagen, are generally the most abundant. They are strong and flexible, yet able to resist stretch. They may be fine or coarse, and they are characteristically unbranched and somewhat wavy. In tissues stained with H&E, they appear pink and refractile. **Reticular fibers** are also formed from the protein collagen. They are delicate, branching fibers that possess a coat of glycoproteins and proteoglycans. They are argyrophilic (silver-loving) and can be stained with silver to distinguish them from other fibers of the connective tissue. They may also be selectively stained with Schiff's reagent. **Elastic fibers,** formed from the protein elastin, range in diameter from fine to coarse and ordinarily cannot be distinguished from collagenous fibers without the use of special stains such as orcein or Weigert's resorcin fuchsin. In some H&E preparations, however, they become colored more intensely by eosin than the collagenous fibers from which they can therefore readily be distinguished. **Fibroblasts** are generally the most numerous of the cells found in connective tissue. They are responsible for the formation of both fibers and ground substance. **Macrophages** (histiocytes), derivatives of monocytes of the blood, are also common inhabitants of connective tissue. They are phagocytic cells that can often be recognized by the presence of debris in their cytoplasm, which gives them a dirty appearance. Other migrants from the blood that are found in connective tissue are **neutrophils** and **eosinophils. Plasma cells, lymphocytes, adipocytes, mast cells,** and globular leukocytes also occur in varying numbers in connective tissue.

All connective tissues are classified on the basis of the arrangement and proportions of their cellular and intercellular components. **Connective tissue proper** includes the general types of connective tissue, loose and dense, as well as the special types, reticular, elastic, and adipose. Mesenchyme and mucous connective tissue are classified as **embryonal connective tissues.**

In **loose** (areolar) **connective tissue,** the ground substance predominates. It contains many scattered cells of various types, vessels, and a loose network of fine collagenous, reticular, and elastic fibers. Loose connective tissue is widespread throughout the body. It surrounds vessels and nerves. It is found in serous membranes such as mesenteries, the lamina propria of mucous membranes, subcutaneous tissue, and the papillary (superficial) layer of the dermis, as well as other places.

In contrast to loose connective tissue, dense connective tissue (often called fibrous tissue) is composed principally of thick collagenous fibers. It contains fewer cells than loose connective tissue, most of which are fibroblasts. In **dense irregular connective tissue,** the collagenous fibers course in all directions, forming a compact three-dimensional meshwork. **Dense regular connective tissue** is characterized by closely packed, parallel bundles of collagenous fibers. Dense irregular connective tissue occurs in such places as the reticular (deep) layer of the dermis, the submucosa of the digestive tract of some species, and the capsules of organs. Tendons, ligaments, and aponeuroses are formed by dense regular connective tissue.

It is helpful to know that there are no sharp lines of distinction between loose and dense irregular connective tissue, or between dense irregular and regular connective tissue. It is not always possible therefore to classify these types of connective tissues with great precision.

Reticular tissue is composed of numerous reticular fibers. It forms a supportive network for the parenchyma of structures such as the spleen, lymph node, liver, kidney, and bone marrow.

Elastic tissue is characterized by numerous regularly or irregularly arranged elastic fibers. It is exemplified by the ligamentum nuchae of grazing animals and by the vocal ligaments.

Adipose tissue consists of groups of adipocytes (also called adipose cells or fat cells) within the loose connective tissue of such places as mesenteries, subcutis, and sheaths of vessels and nerves.

Mesenchyme tissue is found in the embryo. It consists of a loose arrangement of pale, star-shaped (stellate) cells with interconnecting cytoplasmic processes. The mesenchyme cells are embedded in a jellylike, amorphous, ground substance that accumulates fine fibers as development progresses.

Mucous connective tissue, another type of embryonal connective tissue, surrounds the vessels of the umbilical cord. It also occurs in limited regions in adult animals, for instance, the dermis of the comb and wattle of the chicken. It is composed of fibroblasts and loosely arranged, fine, collagenous fibers in an abundant, amorphous ground substance.

Figure 3.1 ×250

Figure 3.2 ×125

Figure 3.3 ×250

Figure 3.4 ×625

Figure 3.5 ×625

KEY	
1. Amorphous ground substance	7. Fibroblast nucleus
2. Collagenous fiber	8. Lymphocyte
3. Elastic fiber	9. Mast cell
4. Eosinophil	10. Mesenchyme cell
5. Epithelium, lip	11. Neutrophil
6. Erythrocytes in capillary	12. Plasma cell

Figure 3.1. Mesenchyme, 72-Hour Embryo, Chicken. Mesenchyme consists of stellate cells. Their processes touch, forming a three-dimensional latticework. The cells are surrounded by an amorphous ground substance.

Figure 3.2. Mucous Connective Tissue, Umbilical Cord, Cow. Mucous connective tissue consists of a loose framework of fibroblasts and collagenous fibers in an amorphous ground substance. Mucous connective tissue of the umbilical cord is often called Wharton's jelly.

Figure 3.3. Loose Connective Tissue, Mesentery, Cat (LeukoStat and Orcein). The loose arrangement of the connective-tissue cells and fibers in this whole mount preparation is evident. Fine, branching elastic fibers appear blue-gray. The thicker, collagenous fibers stain pale pink. Note the mast cell filled with purple granules.

Figure 3.4. Plasma Cells, Loose Connective Tissue, Lamina Propria, Jejunum, Dog. Plasma cells are common constituents of the lamina propria of the gastrointestinal tract. They are characterized by a basophilic cytoplasm and large blocks of nuclear heterochromatin. A lightly stained area adjacent to the usually eccentric nucleus marks the location of the Golgi apparatus.

Figure 3.5. Mast Cells, Loose Connective Tissue, Lip, Cat, (Toluidine Blue). The granules of mast cells are metachromatic and are colored purple by toluidine blue.

Figure 3.6

× 520

KEY		
1. Collagenous fiber	5. Lymphocyte	
2. Eosinophil	6. Mast cell	
3. Fibroblast nucleus	7. Plasma cell	
4. Globular leukocyte		

Figure 3.6. Loose Connective Tissue, Lamina propria, Duodenum, Cow. A loose meshwork of fibers of the connective tissue and various cells are contained in an amorphous, ground substance.

Figure 3.7   × 250

Figure 3.10   × 62.5

Figure 3.8   × 180

KEY	
1. Adipocyte	7. Fibroblast nucleus
2. Arteriole	8. Loose connective tissue
3. Collagenous fiber	9. Macrophage
4. Dense irregular connective tissue	10. Tendon, l.s.
5. Eosinophil	11. Tendon, x.s.
6. Epithelium, planum	

Figure 3.7. Macrophages, Loose Connective Tissue, Colon, Pig. Wandering macrophages are characterized by their oval shape. The cytoplasm of these cells often contains ingested particles and appears dirty. Eosinophils of the pig contain oval or bilobed nuclei.

Figure 3.8. Loose and Dense Irregular Connective Tissue, Dermis, Planum Nasolabiale, Cow. Note that the loose connective tissue of the papillary layer of the dermis contains finer fibers and more cells than the dense irregular connective tissue of the reticular layer.

Figure 3.9. Dense Irregular Connective Tissue, Dermis, Horse. Note the coarse, interwoven, collagenous fibers.

Figure 3.10. Dense Regular Connective Tissue, Tendon, x.s. and l.s., Nose, Pig. In tendons and ligaments, collagenous fibers are arranged in parallel order. Fibroblasts are located between the fibers.

Figure 3.9   × 62.5

Figure 3.11 × 125

Figure 3.15 × 62.5

Figure 3.12 × 62.5

Figure 3.13 × 62.5

Figure 3.14 × 250

KEY	
1. Adipocyte	5. Reticular fiber
2. Elastic fiber	6. Tendon, x.s.
3. Fibroblast nucleus	7. Tendon sheath, inner
4. Lymphocyte	8. Tendon sheath, outer

Figure 3.11. Tendon and Tendon Sheath, x.s., Dog. The tendon sheath is actually made up of two sheaths. The inner sheath attaches to the surface of the tendon. The outer sheath forms a tube around the tendon and attaches to peripheral structures. The space between the two sheaths is filled with synovial fluid in living tissue. The space is not lined by an epithelium, but rather by collagenous fibers and cells of the connective tissue of the sheaths.

Figure 3.12. Elastic Tissue, Ligamentum Nuchae, l.s., Sheep. This section shows the parallel arrangement of the elastic fibers within the ligament.

Figure 3.13. Elastic Tissue, Ligamentum Nuchae, x.s., Sheep, (Orcein). Orcein selectively stains elastic fibers red.

Figure 3.14. Reticular Tissue, Lymph Node, Cow (Silver). Networks of reticular fibers have been blackened by silver.

Figure 3.15. Adipose Tissue, Soft Palate, Cow. Lipid content of each adipocyte (unilocular) was removed during processing, leaving an empty cavity surrounded by a thin rim of cytoplasm. Nuclei occur at the periphery of adipocytes. It is sometimes difficult to distinguish their nuclei from those of other cells of the connective tissue. See Figure 12.104 for an example of multilocular adipocytes.

4

CARTILAGE

Cartilage is a form of connective tissue. There are three basic types of cartilage: **hyaline, elastic,** and **fibrous** (fibrocartilage). Each consists of chondrocytes embedded in an amorphous, ground substance (matrix), which is rich in sulfated glycosaminoglycans complexed with protein to form macromolecules called proteoglycans. The latter are bound electrostatically to unit fibrils of collagen. The matrix is firm but flexible.

Hyaline cartilage is the most common type. It forms large parts of the developing vertebrate skeleton, and it is also found in epiphyseal discs, articular cartilages, the trachea, bronchi, and elsewhere. Its ground substance is separable into pale and darkly stained areas called **interterritorial** and **territorial matrix,** respectively. The higher concentration of sulfated glycosaminoglycans in the latter is responsible for the darker staining. Chondrocytes are confined to small spaces (**lacunae**) within the matrix. Small clusters of chondrocytes, called **isogenous groups,** are frequently observed. They are the result of cell division of chondrocytes. Cartilage matrix is usually invested by a **perichondrium** whose inner layer is chondrogenic, containing cells with the capacity to become chondroblasts. Its outer portion is dense irregular connective tissue.

Elastic cartilage is similar in structure to hyaline cartilage. Its name derives from the presence of large amounts of elastic fibers embedded in the matrix. Among other places, it is found in the epiglottis, parts of the larynx, and the pinna.

Fibrous cartilage is unlike either of the other types. It is dense connective tissue within which are distributed linear groupings of chondrocytes embedded in a small amount of matrix. Fibrous cartilage is found in such places as the intervertebral discs and cardiac skeleton, as well as within some tendons close to their attachment to bone.

Figure 4.1   × 125

Figure 4.2   × 250

Figure 4.3   × 125

Figure 4.4   × 125

Figure 4.5   × 125

KEY	
1. Chondrocyte	6. Matrix
2. Chondrocyte in lacuna	7. Perichondrium, chondrogenic
3. Collagenous fiber	8. Perichondrium, fibrous
4. Elastic fiber	9. Territorial matrix
5. Interterritorial matrix	

Figure 4.1. Hyaline Cartilage, Trachea, Cow. The perichondrium consists of an outer fibrous and an inner chondrogenic layer. Isogenous groups and single chondrocytes are scattered throughout the matrix.

Figure 4.2. Elastic Cartilage, Epiglottis, Dog. Pink elastic fibers can be seen throughout the cartilage matrix.

Figure 4.3. Elastic Cartilage, Wattle, Pig (Orcein). The elastic fibers are stained red with orcein.

Figure 4.4. Fibrocartilage, Intervertebral Disc, Horse. Chondrocytes are arranged in rows and framed by a hazy rim of pale blue matrix. Collagenous fibers are visible between rows of chondrocytes.

Figure 4.5. Fibrocartilage, Claw, Chicken. Rows of chondrocytes are randomly scattered among collagenous fibers. Pale blue matrix is visible around some chondrocytes.

5

BONE

Bone is a living, dynamic connective tissue. Its hardness and strength are provided by a matrix consisting of hydroxyapatites and collagen, respectively. It is admirably suited to its function as a skeletal substance because of its high tensile strength and relatively light weight.

The structure of bone is unrelated to its mode of development; that is, the **lamellae** of **intramembranous bone** have the same basic structure as those of **endochondral (intracartilaginous) bone. Mature bone,** however, contains fewer osteocytes than the **immature bone** it replaces. The woven form of the latter contains numerous osteocytes and an organic matrix of interlacing collagenous fibers. Its matrix has a bluish cast in preparations stained with hematoxylin and eosin. In contrast, the matrix of mature bone is uniformly acidophilic.

Deposits of matrix may be dense, with few spaces between matrix elements (**compact bone**), or they may be in the form of delicate three-dimensional latticeworks (**spongy bone**). Compact bone forms the outer shells of the diaphysis and epiphysis, while spongy bone occurs in the interior of the epiphysis and the endosteal surface of portions of the diaphysis. In the compact bone of the diaphysis, matrix appears as **haversian systems, interstitial systems,** and **circumferential lamellae.**

Although **osteocytes** are entrapped within matrix, they are able to communicate physically through **canaliculi,** which connect lacunae with each other. **Osteoblasts** and **osteoclasts** lie free on the external surface of the matrix. The former secrete most of the matrix and eventually become surrounded by it. They are then called osteocytes. Osteoclasts, large multinucleate cells derived from monocytes, resorb matrix during bone remodeling or when the need for serum calcium arises.

Bone matrix undergoes remarkable transformations in size and shape during development. This process of bone remodeling is especially well exemplified during the formation of the skull and long bones. In both instances, transformations in shape and increases in size are accomplished through the processes of bone deposition and bone resorption.

An important aspect of the growth in length of long bones is the persistence of functional epiphyseal discs. These plates of hyaline cartilage permit the process of intracartilaginous ossification to continue until full growth of the bone is achieved, at which time the discs become replaced by bone and no further lengthening is possible.

Figure 5.1   × 62.5

Figure 5.5   × 25

Figure 5.2   × 250

KEY		
1. Bone marrow	8.	Osteoblast
2. Bone matrix	9.	Osteoclast
3. Calcified cartilage	10.	Osteocyte
4. Epiphyseal disc (plate)	11.	Osteoid
5. Hyaline cartilage	12.	Spongy bone, diaphysis
6. Immature bone	13.	Spongy bone, epiphysis
7. Mature bone		

Figure 5.1. Membrane Bone, Decalcified, Nose, Dog. Osteoblasts deposit bone matrix directly within mesenchyme without a preformed cartilage model. Therefore, the trabeculae of membrane bone lack calcified cartilage cores.

Figure 5.2. Membrane Bone, Decalcified, Nose, Dog (Masson's). Osteoclasts are large, multinucleated giant cells.

Figure 5.3. Immature Bone, Phalanx, Decalcified, Fetus, Horse. Immature bone is characterized by a larger number of osteocytes per unit area than are found in mature bone. Typically, it also shows basophilia. Both characteristics are evident in the micrograph. Note the rather even acidophilia of the matrix of the more mature bone.

Figure 5.4. Primary Center of Ossification, Phalanx, l.s., Decalcified, Fetus, Horse. Section was taken from the central region of a developing phalanx and shows early endochondral ossification.

Figure 5.5. Epiphyseal Disc, Humerus, l.s., Decalcified, Cat. The cartilaginous epiphyseal disc (plate) lies between the spongy bone of the epiphysis and the diaphysis. Also see Figure 5.6.

Figure 5.3   × 62.5

Figure 5.4   × 25

Figure 5.6   × 130

KEY	
1. Bone marrow	7. Spongy bone, epiphysis
2. Bone matrix	8. Zone of calcification
3. Calcified cartilage matrix	9. Zone of hypertrophy
4. Osteoblast	10. Zone of multiplication
5. Osteocyte	11. Zone of ossification
6. Spongy bone, diaphysis	12. Zone of reserve cartilage

Figure 5.6. Epiphyseal Disc, Humerus, l.s., Decalcified, Cat. Various zones of endochondral bone formation. Small, scattered cartilage cells comprise the zone of reserve (resting) cartilage. They proliferate, forming rows that constitute the zone of multiplication (zone of proliferation). The cells then enlarge (zone of hypertrophy). The remaining cartilage matrix between the hypertrophied cells becomes impregnated with calcium salts (zone of calcification). Osteoblasts deposit bone matrix *(pink)* onto the calcified cartilage matrix *(lavender)* in the zone of ossification.

Figure 5.7   × 62.5

Figure 5.8   × 62.5

Figure 5.9   × 125

Figure 5.10   × 280

Figure 5.11   × 125

KEY		
1. Bone marrow	10.	Osteoblast
2. Bone matrix	11.	Osteoclast
3. Calcified cartilage matrix	12.	Osteocyte
4. Canaliculi	13.	Sinusoid
5. Haversian canal	14.	Volkmann's canal
6. Haversian system	15.	Zone of calcification
7. Inner circumferential lamellae	16.	Zone of hypertrophy
8. Interstitial system	17.	Zone of multiplication
9. Lacuna	18.	Zone of ossification

Figure 5.7. Endochondral Bone, Phalanx, l.s., Decalcified, Dog. The zones of calcification and ossification are distinct in this preparation. Calcified cartilage stains an intense purple, while bone matrix is strongly eosinophilic.

Figure 5.8. Endochondral Bone, Epiphysis of Radius, Decalcified, Dog. Spicules of bone *(pink)* with calcified cartilage cores *(lavender)*.

Figure 5.9. Compact Ground Bone, Femur, x.s., Cat (Unstained). A haversian canal surrounded by concentric bony lamellae constitutes a haversian system (osteon). Lacunae with canaliculi (web-like, fine, dark lines) are occupied by osteocytes and their processes, respectively, in living tissue. Volkmann's canals, inner circumferential lamellae, and parts of old haversian systems, called interstitial systems, are present.

Figure 5.10. Compact Ground Long Bone, x.s., Cat (Unstained). The spider web-like channels called canaliculi can be seen surrounding the lacunae.

Figure 5.11. Compact Bone, Humerus, x.s., Decalcified, Chicken. In decalcified bone, hydroxyapatites have been removed, leaving the collagenous portion of the matrix. Blood vessels, osteocytes, and other tissue elements are also left intact. Compare with Figure 5.9.

Figure 5.12   × 125

Figure 5.13   × 62.5

Figure 5.14   × 625

Figure 5.15   × 70

Figure 5.16   × 280

KEY	
1. Artery	8. Osteocyte
2. Endosteum	9. Osteogenic layer, periosteum
3. Fibrous layer, periosteum	10. Periosteum
4. Haversian canal	11. Sharpey's fibers
5. Marrow cavity	12. Tendon
6. Megakaryocyte	13. Vein
7. Nerve	14. Volkmann's canal

Figure 5.12. Compact Bone, x.s., Jaw, Decalcified, Dog. Blood vessels and nerves are evident in this cross section of a haversian canal.

Figure 5.13. Compact Bone, Rib, l.s., Decalcified, Cat. Portions of haversian canals are oriented parallel to the long axis of the bone. The collagenous fibers of a tendon extend into the bone as Sharpey's fibers. The large cells in the bone marrow are megakaryocytes.

Figure 5.14. Compact bone, rib, l.s., Decalcified, Cat. Flat cells of the endosteum line the marrow cavity.

Figure 5.15. Periosteum of femur, l.s., Decalcified, Cat. The periosteum parallels the bone of the diaphysis.

Figure 5.16. Periosteum of femur, l.s., Decalcified, Cat. A magnified view of the periosteum seen in Figure 5.15. The osteogenic layer of the periosteum abuts the bone and is more cellular than the outer fibrous layer of the periosteum.

Figure 5.17   × 62.5

Figure 5.18   × 125

Figure 5.19   × 25

KEY		
1. Articulating surface, P2	6.	Fibrous capsule
2. Articulating surface, P3	7.	Joint cavity
3. Bone matrix	8.	Sharpey's fibers
4. Cartilage	9.	Synovial fold
5. Extensor tendon	10.	Tendon

Figure 5.17. Sharpey's Fibers, Phalanx, l.s., Decalcified, Fetus, Sheep (Mallory's). Collagenous fibers of a tendon become embedded within the bone matrix, where they are called Sharpey's fibers.

Figure 5.18. Sharpey's Fibers, Phalanx, l.s., Decalcified, Fetus, Sheep (Mallory's). Same as Figure 5.17, but magnification has been increased to show the relationship between the bone matrix and the collagenous fibers of the tendon.

Figure 5.19. Distal Interphalangeal Joint, l.s., Fetus, Horse. The mid-dorsal aspect of this developing synovial joint is shown. The joint capsule is composed of a fibrous portion and a well-vascularized, synovial membrane. The latter lines the joint cavity, except for the articulating surfaces. Synovial folds project into the cavity. The outer, more fibrous portion of the capsule is continuous with the future periosteum of the phalanges and blends dorsally with the extensor tendon. The tendon is attached to the developing extensor process of P_3. Note that the phalanges have not yet begun to ossify. After ossification, a layer of hyaline cartilage will persist on the articular surfaces.

6

BLOOD

Blood is a special type of connective tissue composed of formed elements in a fluid matrix. **Plasma** is the fluid portion, called **serum** when depleted of fibrinogen. The **formed elements** include erythrocytes (red blood cells), leukocytes (white blood cells), and platelets (thrombocytes in birds).

Blood cells and platelets are usually examined in stained blood smears (blood films). To make such a preparation, a drop of blood is spread thinly on a glass slide, dried, and stained with a Romanovsky-type stain such as Giemsa or Wright's. One end of the film is usually much thinner than the other end. Details of cell morphology are more visible in the thin film, where the cells are more flattened and less crowded. Blood smears should be scanned with the high-dry objective. With practice, most cells can be differentiated at this magnification. Oil immersion should be reserved for studying specific cells in more detail.

MAMMALS

Mature **erythrocytes** are small, anucleate cells uniquely adapted to transport oxygen and carbon dioxide to and from tissues. They are acidophilic and acquire an orange to red color with Romanovsky stains.

The average diameter of erythrocytes in a dried smear varies with the species. The erythrocytes of the dog are largest (7.0 μm), while those of the goat are the smallest (4.1 μm). Red blood cells from the same animal are all approximately the same size except in the cow, where variation in the size of the erythrocytes (anisocytosis) is not unusual. In most species the cells are disc-shaped, although in young goats they may also be angulated.

Central pallor, resulting from its biconcave shape, is best defined in the erythrocyte of the dog, but may be seen in other domestic mammals. Red blood cells sometimes adhere to each other, forming an arrangement resembling a stack of coins, called a rouleaux. This occurs commonly in the horse and cat. It is rare in ruminants. Crenated erythrocytes, characterized by pointed cell margins, are observed most often in pigs.

Various factors influence the appearance of red (and white) blood cells. These include the freshness of the blood sample, the use of an anticoagulant, how quickly the smear was dried, and the thickness of the smear. The occurrence of central pallor, rouleaux, and crenation varies not only with the species, but also with each smear and within different regions of the same smear.

Leukocytes are basic cellular components of the immune system. They are nucleated cells that are larger and less numerous than erythrocytes. They are classified, depending on the presence or absence of specific cytoplasmic granules, as either **granulocytes** (neutrophils, eosinophils, and basophils) or **agranulocytes** (lymphocytes and monocytes). Leukocytes tend to accumulate along the edges of a blood smear, so that examples of them, although often distorted, can be found more readily in these regions.

Lymphocytes are the predominant leukocytes in ruminants and pigs. The cells range in size from 6 to 15 μm and are sometimes classified as small, medium, and large. Most of the lymphocytes in carnivores, horses, and pigs are small. Larger cells occur more often in ruminants.

Small lymphocytes have a relatively large, dense, often eccentric nucleus that is round and may be slightly indented. In the cat the nucleus is sometimes deeply indented like a kidney. The nucleus tends to be oval in the pig. Some of the lymphocytes of ruminants are binucleate.

Only a thin rim of cytoplasm may be visible in the small lymphocyte. The cytoplasm is basophilic and may show a lighter region (perinuclear halo) adjacent to the nucleus. At times, nonspecific azurophilic granules may be seen in the cytoplasm of both small and large lymphocytes.

A large lymphocyte has a less dense nucleus and paler, more abundant cytoplasm than a small lymphocyte. The nucleus may be round, oval, or kidney-shaped.

Monocytes are the largest of the leukocytes (15 to 20 μm in diameter). The nuclear chromatin tends to be diffuse, appearing lacy or sometimes patchy. The shape of the nucleus is highly variable and may be oval, irregular, kidney-shaped, or horseshoe-shaped. In the horse the nucleus is frequently kidney-shaped. In ruminants the nucleus may appear amoeboid and sometimes has a three-pronged configuration or is shaped like a cloverleaf.

The cytoplasm is generally pale gray-blue and may contain dustlike, azurophilic granules. It often contains vacuoles that give it a foamy appearance. In ruminants the cytoplasm can be more basophilic and either granular or mottled in appearance.

Neutrophils are the predominant leukocytes in the dog, cat, and horse. The dark-staining nucleus of the mature cell contains very densely packed chromatin. It is long and narrow and may be monolobed or segmented. The nucleus is sometimes coiled, as it is in the cat and, more often, in the pig. When segmented, the lobes may be separated by slight indentations or thin strands of nucleoplasm. The nuclear membrane may appear irregular or tattered from bulging clumps of chromatin. In the horse the chromatin is so heavily clumped that the nucleus appears very jagged.

The pale gray cytoplasm of the neutrophil contains pink, dustlike, specific granules that may be difficult to resolve with the light microscope. The granules are smallest in the dog, so that the cytoplasm appears nongranular and very faint. Granulation is most pronounced in the sheep and goat. In these animals larger, more darkly stained granules occur among the finer pink granules.

Band forms of the neutrophil (and other granulocytes) may be encountered in a smear of peripheral blood. The nucleus of these cells looks like a curved or U-shaped band. It can be distinguished from a mature, monolobed granulocyte by the relatively smooth, rather than ragged, contour of the nucleus. Also, the chromatin is less condensed, and the nucleus appears paler and plumper than in the mature cell.

The nucleus of the **eosinophil,** although similar to that of the neutrophil, tends to be less dense and have fewer lobes. In the pig the nucleus is commonly oval or kidney-shaped rather than segmented. C-shaped, monolobed nuclei are common in ruminants.

The cytoplasm of the eosinophil stains pale blue or gray. Specific granules stain various shades of orange, pink, or red with eosin. The granules of the eosinophil of the dog, unlike those of other domestic mammals, are highly variable in size and do not usually fill the cell. Occasionally, small, clear vacuoles also occur in the cytoplasm. In the cat the granules are rod-shaped. Large, round to oblong granules are a striking feature of the eosinophil of the horse. They usually fill the cytoplasm and cause the cell membrane to bulge, so that the eosinophil resembles a raspberry. In the pig, sheep, and goat the granules are small, round to oval, and numerous, often distorting the cell membrane. In cows the granules are round and intensely stained.

Only a small percentage (0.5 to 3%) of the leukocytes of domestic mammals are **basophils.** Hence, they are not often found in blood smears. The basophil nucleus may be irregular, bilobed, or highly segmented. The granules of basophils vary in size, number, and staining intensity. They are often fairly large, round to oval, and stain reddish purple to dark purple. The granules are a dumbbell or coccoid shape in the pig. The basophil of the cat is much different from that of the other domestic mammals. The granules are small and not deeply stained. They are dull gray to lavender in a lavender cytoplasm.

Because the nuclei of the granulocytes exhibit many forms, the cells are also called **polymorphonuclear leukocytes** (polymorphs, PMNs). These terms, however, are sometimes used specifically as synonyms for the neutrophil.

Platelets play an important role in hemostasis. Although also referred to as thrombocytes, they are not cells. They are membrane-bound fragments of cytoplasm from large cells called megakaryocytes, found in the bone marrow and sometimes the lymph nodes and spleen. Platelets are small and pale blue, and they have purple central granules in stained smears. They occur singly or in clusters in smears of peripheral blood.

CHICKEN

Mature **erythrocytes** of the chicken are very different from those of domestic mammals. They are large, elongated, flat cells with an oval nucleus. In dried blood smears from White Leghorn chickens, they range from approximately 9 to 12 μm long and 6 to 8 μm wide. Their size varies with the breed and the sex of the bird. The nucleus contains small, uniformly distributed clumps of chromatin. The cytoplasm stains a pale orange to pink color.

Thrombocytes are nucleated cells, related in function to the platelets of mammals. They are smaller and less elongated than erythrocytes and have a larger, more round nucleus. The pale, dull blue cytoplasm is characterized by one or more small magenta granules and vacuoles.

Lymphocytes are the most numerous of the leukocytes in the chicken. Their size varies from small to large, as in mammals. The cytoplasm is slightly basophilic and may appear granular or homogeneous. The nucleus is round, sometimes slightly indented, and usually centrally located. The chromatin occurs in coarse clumps, except in the larger lymphocytes where it is finer.

Monocytes are usually larger than lymphocytes. The nuclear chromatin tends to be more diffuse. Vacuoles are often seen in the cytoplasm.

Heterophils are the most abundant of the granulocytes. Both heterophils and eosinophils have acidophilic, specific granules. The granules of the heterophil are rod-shaped or spindle-shaped. Their centers sometimes contain a distinctive, ruby red, spheric granule. During staining there may be partial or complete dissolution of the rods, leaving only the more stable, central granule. The granules of the **eosinophil** are round and pink. Its cytoplasm is pale blue, in contrast to the clear cytoplasm of the heterophil. In both of these granulocytes the nucleus is polymorphic. In the eosinophil the nucleus generally has fewer lobes and also exhibits dense blocks of chromatin clearly separated by lighter areas. This contrasts with the less distinctly clumped chromatin of the heterophil.

The **basophils** of the chicken are much more numerous than in mammals. Their specific granules are deeply basophilic, and the nucleus is usually unlobed and pale.

Figure 6.1   × 312

Figure 6.2   × 781

Figure 6.3   × 781

Figure 6.4   × 781

Figure 6.5   × 781

KEY	
1. Basophil	7. Neutrophil
2. Eosinophil	8. Plasma
3. Erythrocyte	9. Platelet
4. Leukocyte	10. Smudged eosinophil
5. Lymphocyte, small	11. Stain precipitate
6. Monocyte	

Figure 6.1. Blood Cells in Section, Artery, Cat. Biconcave, disc-shaped red blood cells, leukocytes, and plasma (pale pink) are within the lumen of an artery.

Figure 6.2. Blood, Dog (Giemsa). The cytoplasm of the monocyte is, typically, vacuolated. The nucleus is frequently oval or U-shaped. Central pallor of the erythrocytes in this preparation is evident.

Figure 6.3. Blood, Dog (Giemsa). The cytoplasm of the small lymphocyte is very sparse and the nuclear chromatin is condensed. The mature neutrophil has a polymorphic nucleus. The pale cytoplasm, barely discernible, is a characteristic of the neutrophil of the dog.

Figure 6.4. Blood, Dog (Giemsa). The basophil has a polymorphic nucleus and coarse granules of various sizes.

Figure 6.5. Blood, Dog (Giemsa). In the eosinophil of the dog, the granules vary in size and number. Vacuoles occur in the cytoplasm. The eosinophil on the right is partially smudged.

Figure 6.6   × 312

Figure 6.7   × 781

Figure 6.8   × 781

Figure 6.9   × 312

Figure 6.10   × 781

KEY		
1. Basophil	4.	Monocyte
2. Eosinophil	5.	Neutrophil
3. Lymphocyte, medium	6.	Platelet

Figure 6.6. Blood, Cat (Giemsa). Eosinophil, neutrophil, lymphocyte, and monocyte.

Figure 6.7. Blood, Cat (Giemsa). Two monocytes. Red cells are stacked in rouleaux.

Figure 6.8. Buffy Coat, Cat (Giemsa). Two eosinophils, one neutrophil, one basophil, and platelets are visible. Eosinophils of the cat have pink, rod-shaped granules. The cytoplasm of the basophil contains numerous, small, round, lavender granules that are tightly packed and may be difficult to resolve. Distinct red granules are scattered among the lavender granules.

Figure 6.9. Blood, Horse (Giemsa). Eosinophil, monocyte, neutrophil, and lymphocyte are visible. In the neutrophil of the horse, the nucleus often appears very jagged.

Figure 6.10. Blood, Horse (Giemsa). A typical monocyte with pale cytoplasm and linearly arranged chromatin.

Figure 6.11   × 781

Figure 6.15   × 781

KEY		
1. Basophil	6.	Lymphocyte, small
2. Basophil granules	7.	Monocyte
3. Eosinophil	8.	Neutrophil
4. Erythrocyte, crenated	9.	Platelet
5. Lymphocyte, large	10.	Smudged cell

Figure 6.12   × 781

Figure 6.11. Blood, Horse (Giemsa). The eosinophil of the horse has characteristic, large, round granules. The surface of the cell appears bumpy where granules are pressed against the plasma membrane, giving the cell a raspberry-like appearance. Note the rouleaux, which are common in the horse.

Figure 6.12. Buffy Coat, Horse (Giemsa). Basophil and neutrophil. Granules of the basophil are purple and vary in size and shape.

Figure 6.13. Blood, Pig (Giemsa). Two large lymphocytes and a monocyte.

Figure 6.14. Blood, Pig (Giemsa). Two lymphocytes, one neutrophil, and two eosinophils. The eosinophil of the pig contains numerous pink, round granules that fill the cytoplasm completely. The nucleus of the eosinophil is not highly segmented. It varies from oval to kidney-shaped. Note the coiled appearance of the nucleus of the neutrophil, a common feature in pigs and cats. Crenated red blood cells are commonly seen in blood smears from the pig. Rouleaux are also evident in this field.

Figure 6.15. Blood, Pig (Giemsa). Eosinophil, basophil, and smudged cell. The granules of the basophil of the pig are dumbbell or coccoid in shape. Some of the granules have been squeezed from the basophil in this preparation.

Figure 6.13   × 781

Figure 6.14   × 781

Figure 6.16   × 781

Figure 6.20   × 781

Figure 6.17   × 625

Figure 6.16. Blood, Cow (Giemsa). Medium lymphocyte and monocyte. The cytoplasm of the monocyte is darker and more granular than that of the lymphocyte.

Figure 6.17. Blood, Cow (Giemsa). Large lymphocyte and neutrophil. Large lymphocytes of the cow often show a deeply indented nucleus. Their cytoplasm is granular and vacuolated.

Figure 6.18. Blood, Cow (Giemsa). The red granules of the eosinophil are small, round, and intensely stained in the cow. The nucleus may be lobed, but is usually C-shaped.

Figure 6.19. Blood, Sheep (Giemsa). The nucleus of the monocytes of ruminants may be oval, indented, or trilobed. The cytoplasm is gray-blue and vacuolated and may contain granules.

Figure 6.20. Blood, Sheep (Giemsa). Monocyte with trilobed nucleus. Compare with Figure 6.19. Our observations have revealed that some monocytes with trilobed nuclei occur in cows and goats also.

Figure 6.18   × 781

Figure 6.19   × 781

Figure 6.21   × 781

Figure 6.25   × 781

Figure 6.22   × 781

KEY	
1. Azurophilic granules	5. Lymphocyte, medium
2. Eosinophil	6. Lymphocyte, small
3. Lymphocyte, binucleate	7. Neutrophil
4. Lymphocyte, large	8. Platelet

Figure 6.21. Blood, Sheep (Giemsa). Lymphocyte with azurophilic granules.

Figure 6.22. Blood, Sheep (Giemsa). Lymphocyte and neutrophil. The cytoplasm of the neutrophil of sheep and goats contains numerous small and a few large, pink granules. A perinuclear halo is commonly seen around the periphery of the nucleus of lymphocytes.

Figure 6.23. Blood, Sheep (Giemsa). The eosinophil of the sheep contains pink, densely packed, oval granules that are uniform in size.

Figure 6.24. Blood, Goat (Giemsa). A lymphocyte and a neutrophil. The chromatin of the lymphocyte is in the form of closely apposed clumps. Granules are evident in the cytoplasm of the neutrophil.

Figure 6.25. Buffy Coat, Goat (Giemsa). Some lymphocytes of the cow, sheep, and goat are binucleate.

Figure 6.23   × 781

Figure 6.24   × 781

Figure 6.26   × 625

Figure 6.30   × 781

Figure 6.27   × 781

KEY	
1. Eosinophil	6. Monocyte
2. Erythrocyte	7. Neutrophil
3. Granulocyte	8. Thrombocyte
4. Heterophil	9. Vacuole
5. Lymphocyte, large	

Figure 6.26. Buffy Coat, Goat (Giemsa). Lymphocyte, monocyte, and neutrophil. The cytoplasm of the monocyte is blue and contains vacuoles that are often seen in clusters.

Figure 6.27. Buffy Coat, Goat (Giemsa). The small, round, acidophilic granules of the eosinophil of the goat almost fill the cytoplasm.

Figure 6.28. Blood Cells in Section, Chicken. Elongated, nucleated red blood cells and a few granulocytes are shown in the lumen of a blood vessel.

Figure 6.29. Blood, Chicken (Wright-Giemsa). Erythrocytes, leukocytes, and thrombocytes.

Figure 6.30. Blood, Chicken (Wright-Giemsa). An oval, coarsely granular nucleus and a vacuolated cytoplasm with one or more magenta granules characterize the thrombocyte.

Figure 6.28   × 250

Figure 6.29   × 312

Figure 6.31   × 781

KEY	
1. Basophil	5. Lymphocyte
2. Eosinophil	6. Monocyte
3. Heterophil	7. Smudged heterophil
4. Immature erythrocyte	

Figure 6.31. Blood, Chicken (Wright-Giemsa). Eosinophil, two lymphocytes, and a heterophil. The heterophil has numerous rod-shaped granules. Some of these may show a ruby-red, spheric granule at the center. The nuclear chromatin is coarse and densely packed. In contrast, the eosinophil has fewer, round, pink granules in a pale blue cytoplasm. The nuclear chromatin is blocklike, the blocks being distinctly separated from each other.

Figure 6.32. Blood, Chicken (Wright-Giemsa). Monocyte and heterophil. Many of the rod-shaped granules of the heterophil have a ruby red, spheric granule at their center. This is a common characteristic of the heterophil. The monocyte has a pale, basophilic, and vacuolated cytoplasm.

Figure 6.33. Blood, Chicken (Wright-Giemsa). Basophil, monocyte, and immature erythrocyte. The basophil is characterized by large numbers of medium-size basophilic granules. Unlike other granulocytes, the nucleus of this cell is usually unlobed. The cytoplasm of the immature erythrocyte is more basophilic and the nucleus is less condensed than in a mature erythrocyte.

Figure 6.34. Blood, Chicken (Wright-Giemsa). Eosinophil and smudged heterophil. The rod-shaped granules of the heterophil and the round granules of the eosinophil are clearly visible in this preparation.

Figure 6.32   × 781

Figure 6.33   × 781

Figure 6.34   × 781

7

BONE MARROW

MAMMALS

Red bone marrow is highly cellular and is specialized to produce blood cells and platelets. Along with the spleen and liver, it plays a role in hematopoiesis during prenatal development. At the time of birth it is the principal source of blood cells and is found throughout the entire skeleton of the animal. In the adult, red marrow is mostly limited to the sternum, ribs, vertebrae, skull, ilia, and the ends of long bones. Yellow marrow, rich in adipose tissue, occupies the remainder of the skeleton of an adult.

Red marrow consists of extravascular hematopoietic tissue and vascular sinusoids. The hematopoietic tissue is rich in blood cells in various stages of formation. It also contains cells of the connective tissue and is supported by a reticular meshwork. Pluripotent stem cells provide a source of unipotent stem cells committed to the formation of either erythrocytes, granulocytes, agranulocytes, or megakaryocytes. Generally, immature (early) cells of the bone marrow are relatively large, and they have a euchromatic nucleus with nucleoli. As they divide and mature, the cells become smaller, the nucleus becomes more heterochromatic, and the nucleoli disappear. Older cells predominate over the immature forms.

The progression of cell stages, from the morphologically indistinct stem cell to a specific mature blood cell, comprises a cell series (cell line). Most of the cells seen in preparations of the bone marrow belong to either the erythroid or granulocytic (myeloid) series. The cells of these series are presented in this chapter.

The **proerythrocyte** (rubriblast, proerythroblast) is a large, round cell with a basophilic cytoplasm. The nucleus is large, with finely granular chromatin and a few nucleoli. This cell undergoes several divisions, giving rise to **basophilic erythroblasts** (prorubricytes). These cells are round with round nuclei. They are the earliest cells of the erythroid series that can be readily identified in smears. The basophilic erythroblast is somewhat smaller than its precursor and has a deeply basophilic cytoplasm. The nuclear chromatin is more coarsely clumped, and no nucleoli are visible. Basophilic erythroblasts give rise to polychromatophilic erythroblasts (rubricytes), which are smaller cells. The chromatin is more condensed, appearing as blocks separated by light streaks, similar to the chromatin of a plasma cell. The cytoplasm is mottled with pink and blue areas. As hemoglobin synthesis continues and ribosomes diminish, the cytoplasm becomes more pink and less blue. Mitotic division usually ceases in the late polychromatophilic erythroblast stage. **Orthochromatophilic erythroblasts** (normoblasts, metarubricytes) are characterized by a round, highly condensed, and deeply stained nucleus. Their cytoplasm is distinctly eosinophilic, but may show slight tinges of blue. Eventually, the nucleus is extruded, leaving an anucleate **reticulocyte** that matures into an erythrocyte.

Myeloblasts are large granulocytic cells with a grainy, basophilic cytoplasm. The round to oval nucleus contains finely dispersed chromatin. Nucleoli may be present. These cells give rise to the **promyelocyte,** the earliest stage in the development of a granulocyte that can be readily distinguished in smears. This cell contains a relatively large nucleus with nucleoli and chromatin that is beginning to clump. The cytoplasm contains nonspecific azurophilic (magenta) granules. Promyelocytes divide and give rise to **myelocytes.** The myelocyte is smaller and has an oval, often eccentric, nucleus with more condensed chromatin. Specific granules, characteristic of neutrophils, eosinophils, or basophils, are apparent in the cytoplasm. Late myelocytes lose the capacity to divide. They are known as metamyelocytes when the nucleus becomes indented and more condensed. With further modification the nucleus becomes more elongated in the **band-cell** stage before eventually assuming the shape found in the **mature granulocyte.**

Megakaryocytes are situated in the extravascular compartment, close to sinusoids, into which they release platelets. They are very large cells with a polymorphic nucleus and a grainy cytoplasm, and they are often seen in preparations of the bone marrow together with a variety of other cells such as plasma cells, adipocytes, and cells in mitosis. **Osteoblasts** and **osteoclasts,** which are closely associated with the surface of the bone lining the marrow cavity, may also be encountered in smear preparations of marrow.

CHICKEN

The organization of bone marrow of the chicken is different from that of mammals. Erythropoiesis takes place within the vascular sinusoids, rather than in the extravascular tissue. The immature red blood cells (large cells with a basophilic cytoplasm) are found adjacent to the endothelium of a sinusoid. As division and maturation of these cells progress, the older ones move inward. Thus, mature erythrocytes (with an eosinophilic cytoplasm) accumulate in the center of the vessel. As in mammals, cells of the granulocytic series (heterophils, eosinophils, and basophils) develop in the extravascular spaces of the marrow.

Figure 7.1   × 312

Figure 7.5   × 781

Figure 7.2   × 312

Figure 7.1. Megakaryocyte, Bone Marrow, Cat (Giemsa). The megakaryocyte is a large cell with a polymorphic nucleus and grainy cytoplasm. Blood platelets are derived from fragments of the cytoplasm. Forces generated during the formation of the smear appear to have separated a segment of the nucleus.

Figure 7.2. Osteoclast, Bone Marrow, Cat (Giemsa). The osteoclast is a large, multinucleate cell formed from fused macrophages. Azurophilic bone debris can be seen in the cytoplasm of this specimen.

Figure 7.3. Osteoblasts, Bone Marrow, Cat (Giemsa). Osteoblasts are characterized by the presence of an eccentric nucleus and basophilic cytoplasm. A perinuclear clear zone, representing the site of the Golgi apparatus, may be visible. In smears these cells often occur in clusters.

Figure 7.4. Bone Marrow, Cat (Giemsa). A variety of different cells of the bone marrow can be identified at this magnification.

Figure 7.5. Bone Marrow, Cat (Giemsa). Basophilic and eosinophilic myelocytes are represented in this field.

Figure 7.3   × 312

Figure 7.4   × 312

Figure 7.6   × 781

Figure 7.7   × 781

Figure 7.8   × 781

Figure 7.9   × 781

Figure 7.10   × 781

KEY	
1. Basophilic band cell	9. Neutrophil
2. Basophilic erythroblast	10. Neutrophilic band cell
3. Basophilic myelocyte	11. Neutrophilic metamyelocyte
4. Endothelial cell, nucleus	12. Neutrophilic metamyelocyte, late
5. Eosinophil	13. Orthochromatophilic erythroblast
6. Erythrocyte, early	14. Polychromatophilic erythroblast
7. Erythrocyte, mature	15. Promyelocyte
8. Heterophil	16. Reticulocyte

Figure 7.6. Bone Marrow, Cat (Wright-Giemsa). A basophilic myelocyte, segmented eosinophil, and polychromatophilic erythroblast are evident.

Figure 7.7. Bone Marrow, Cat (Wright-Giemsa). Various myeloid developmental stages are shown in this field.

Figure 7.8. Bone Marrow, Cat (Wright-Giemsa). Various erythroid developmental stages are shown in this field.

Figure 7.9. Bone Marrow, Cat (Wright-Giemsa). The largest cell seen in this field is a promyelocyte. Note the presence of numerous magenta, azurophilic granules in its cytoplasm.

Figure 7.10. Bone Marrow, Plastic Section, Chicken (Giemsa). Intravascular developmental stages of erythrocytes are shown. In the extravascular compartment, heterophils and eosinophils can be distinguished.

8

MUSCLE

A unique characteristic of muscle cells is the presence of a substructure of myofilaments that provides them with the ability to contract. Although the arrangement of the myofilaments in cells of smooth muscle differs from that of cells of skeletal and cardiac muscle, the contraction process is the same. This process occurs when the filaments slide past one another resulting in a shortening of the cell.

Smooth muscle is involuntary. Its cells are long and tapered and have an elongated nucleus located about midway between the ends of each cell. Smooth muscle consists of groups of these cells bound together by connective tissue fibers. Students often encounter difficulty in distinguishing smooth muscle from the surrounding connective tissue. It is helpful to know that smooth muscle presents an overall dull, pink appearance in hematoxylin and eosin preparations, while fibers of the connective tissue are considerably more refractile and appear bright pink and shiny by comparison.

Smooth muscle is found in a variety of places, for example, throughout the digestive tract, in blood vessels, in the urinary bladder, in the capsules of some organs, and in bronchi.

Skeletal muscle is striated and voluntary. Cells are multinucleated and may be 3 or 4 cm long. Cross-striations result from the precise registration of the A, I, H, and M bands of the sarcomeres of the myofibrils. Nuclei are located peripherally, immediately below the sarcolemma. Individual cells are grouped into fascicles. Each fascicle, in turn, is surrounded by a **perimysium** of loose connective tissue. Each cell within a fascicle is closely invested by delicate reticular fibers, the **endomysium.** Groups of fascicles are bound together by a sheath of dense connective tissue, the **epimysium.** Collagenous fibers of tendons insert into invaginations at the ends of the muscle cell, anchoring the tendon to an external lamina, which is adherent to the sarcolemma.

Cardiac muscle is striated and involuntary. It forms the myocardium of the heart and occurs in the walls of the major vessels carrying blood to and from the heart, including the aorta, pulmonary artery, pulmonary vein, and vena cava. A single, centrally located nucleus occurs in most cells. Occasionally, however, a cell with two nuclei may be seen. The cell's cross-striations result from the precise registration of sarcomeric bands as in skeletal muscle. Unlike cells of skeletal or smooth muscle, cells of cardiac muscle branch and anastomose with one another. Special cell-surface modifications called **intercalated discs** join cells of cardiac muscle together end to end.

Some cells of cardiac muscle are modified and function as a conducting system that helps to coordinate the heart beat. These modified cells are the functional elements of the sinoatrial node, atrioventricular node, and the Purkinje fibers.

Figure 8.1   × 250

Figure 8.2   × 250

Figure 8.3   × 180

Figure 8.4   × 62.5

KEY	
1. Arteriole	7. Muscle cell, oblique cut
2. Capillary, x.s.	8. Muscle cell, x.s.
3. Connective tissue	9. Perimysium
4. Endomysium	10. Tendon
5. Muscle cell, l.s.	11. Venule
6. Muscle cell, nucleus	

Figure 8.1. Smooth Muscle, x.s. and l.s., Muscularis Externa, Jejunum, x.s., Sheep. Cells of smooth muscle have a single, elongated nucleus. This is apparent in cells that have been sectioned longitudinally. Cross sections of smooth-muscle cells vary in diameter, depending on where they were transected along their length. If the cell was transected through its middle region, the nucleus is visible and appears round. If the cut was closer to the tapered extremity of the cell, no nucleus is evident and the cell has a smaller diameter.

Figure 8.2. Smooth Muscle, x.s. and l.s., Urinary Bladder, Pig. The tapered form of the smooth-muscle cell is evident.

Figure 8.3. Skeletal Muscle, x.s. and l.s., Tongue, Horse. Cells of skeletal muscle are large and possess numerous, peripheral nuclei. Cross-striations are evident in cells cut longitudinally.

Figure 8.4. Skeletal Muscle and Tendon, oblique cut, Tongue, Horse. The collagenous fibers of a tendon can be seen blending with skeletal-muscle cells.

Figure 8.5

× 1300

Figure 8.5. Skeletal Muscle, l.s., Lip, Dog (Masson's). Portions of two muscle cells showing individual myofibrils and cross-striations.

Figure 8.6   × 625

Figure 8.7   × 125

Figure 8.9   × 625

KEY	
1. Bifurcation	5. Muscle cell, l.s.
2. Capillary, x.s.	6. Muscle cell, nucleus
3. Endomysium	7. Muscle cell, x.s.
4. Intercalated disc	8. Myofibrils

Figure 8.6. Skeletal Muscle, x.s., Tongue, Horse. Transected my-ofibrils can be clearly seen within each cell.

Figure 8.7. Cardiac Muscle, l.s., Heart, Cat. Bifurcations in the cardiac-muscle cells are visible.

Figure 8.8. Cardiac Muscle, l.s., Cat. Cross-striations and inter-calated discs are apparent in this preparation.

Figure 8.9. Cardiac Muscle, x.s., Pig. Note the centrally located nuclei of the muscle cell.

Figure 8.8   × 360

9

NERVOUS SYSTEM

One can hardly examine a histologic preparation of any sort without finding some evidence of nervous tissue, for example, sections through myelinated or unmyelinated nerves, isolated neurons, encapsulated nerve endings, or perhaps a nerve plexus.

The nervous system consists of neurons of various sizes and kinds, including their supporting elements, and is basically similar in all domestic animals. In the central nervous system there is a structural framework provided by neuroglia cells and their processes. Additionally, meninges, formed of connective tissue, surround the brain and spinal cord providing support and protection. In the peripheral nervous system, neuroglia cells are lacking and the system's various components are supported by connective tissue and special cells. For example, axons and bundles of axons of peripheral nerves are fastened together by both loose and dense irregular connective tissue and the processes of neurons are supported by Schwann cells.

Selected examples of nervous system elements as they typically appear in histologic preparations of various kinds are presented. Additionally, sections through portions of the brain, brain stem, and spinal cord have been included. The organs of special sense, the eye and ear, are treated in separate chapters.

Figure 9.1   × 25

Figure 9.5   × 62.5

Figure 9.2   × 125

KEY	
1. Blood vessel	9. Periosteum
2. Bone, skull	10. Pia mater
3. Dendrite	11. Purkinje cell
4. Dura mater	12. Pyramidal cell
5. Granular layer	13. Pyramidal cell layer
6. Mesothelium	14. Subarachnoid space
7. Molecular layer	15. White matter
8. Outer granular layer	

Figure 9.1. Cerebellum, Sheep. The molecular and granular layers of the gray matter and Purkinje cells are shown. The white matter lies deep to the gray matter.

Figure 9.2. Cerebellum, Sheep. Portions of the dendritic tree of the multipolar Purkinje cells are visible.

Figure 9.3. Cerebral Cortex, Dog. Outer portion of cerebral cortex with numerous blood vessels.

Figure 9.4. Cerebral Cortex, Pyramidal Cells, Dog. Magnified view of cells of the pyramidal layer.

Figure 9.5. Dura Mater, Goat. The dura remains attached to the skull when the latter is separated from the brain. It is a dense fibroelastic layer lined by a mesothelium. The dura merges with the periosteum of the skull.

Figure 9.3   × 62.5

Figure 9.4   × 250

Figure 9.6

× 260

KEY	
1. Arachnoid layer	4. Molecular layer
2. Cerebrospinal fluid	5. Pia mater
3. Collagenous fiber	6. Small artery

Figure 9.6. Meninges, Cerebellum, Sheep (Mallory's). The arachnoid layer, subarachnoid space, and pia mater are shown. The subarachnoid space is filled with cerebrospinal fluid, which is stained purple. Wisps of collagenous fibers *(blue)* can be seen within the subarachnoid space. These connect the arachnoid layer with the pia.

Figure 9.7

× 125

Figure 9.11

× 125

Figure 9.8

× 12.5

KEY	
1. Astrocyte, cell body	10. Medulla
2. Astrocyte, process	11. Molecular layer
3. Brain sand	12. Neuron
4. Capillary	13. Perivascular space
5. Cerebellum, vermis	14. Pia mater
6. Choroid plexus	15. Purkinje cell
7. Epithelium	16. Venule
8. Fourth ventricle	17. Villus, x.s.
9. Granular layer	

Figure 9.7. Cerebellum, Dog. Portion of a sulcus containing a venule. The perivascular space surrounding the vessel is continuous with the subarachnoid space and separates the vessel from the pia mater on either side.

Figure 9.8. Choroid Plexus, Cat (Cresyl Violet). Portion of the fourth ventricle with choroid plexus in the roof of the medulla.

Figure 9.9. Choroid Plexus, Dog. The simple cuboidal epithelium and large, thin-walled capillaries are major constituents of the villi of the choroid plexus.

Figure 9.10. Brain Sand, Hypothalamus, Dog. Calcified, granular material called brain sand can be found dispersed through various parts of the brain, including the hypothalamus, cerebellum, and pineal gland.

Figure 9.11. Fibrous Astrocytes, Medulla, Cat (Golgi). These neuroglia cells have long processes that show little or no branching.

Figure 9.9

× 125

Figure 9.10

× 62.5

Figure 9.12

× 26

KEY	
1. Central canal	3. Multipolar neuron
2. Gray matter, ventral horn	4. White matter

Figure 9.12. Spinal Cord, Cervical, x.s., Sheep (Masson's). The central canal, gray matter, and white matter are shown.

Figure 9.13   × 125

Figure 9.16   × 62.5

Figure 9.14   × 125

Figure 9.13. Central Canal, Spinal Cord, x.s., Sheep. Tall ependymal cells, some of which are ciliated, line the central canal.

Figure 9.14. Multipolar Neurons, Spinal Cord, Sheep. The axon hillock of two neurons can be seen. Nissl granules are absent from the hillock region, but extend into the dendrites.

Figure 9.15. Multipolar Neurons, Spinal Cord, Cow. Two multipolar neurons are shown in this smear preparation. Note prominent nucleoli and Nissl granules.

Figure 9.16. Dorsal Root Ganglion, Dog (Luxol Fast Blue/Cresylecht Violet). Portion of a dorsal root ganglion showing neurons and nerve fibers. (Photomicrograph of a histologic section borrowed from the College of Veterinary Medicine, Iowa State University.)

Figure 9.15   × 180

Figure 9.17   × 250

Figure 9.21   × 12.5

Figure 9.18   × 125

KEY	
1. Adipose tissue	8. Neuron cell body
2. Epineurium	9. Nissl granules
3. Muscularis externa, inner circular	10. Perineurium
4. Muscularis externa, outer longitudinal	11. Plexus
5. Muscularis mucosae	12. Satellite cell
6. Nerve	13. Submucosa
7. Nerve fiber	

Figure 9.17. Dorsal Root Ganglion, Dog (Luxol Fast Blue/Cresylecht Violet). Flattened satellite cells envelop the round neuron cell bodies of the unipolar neurons. (Photograph of a histologic section borrowed from the College of Veterinary Medicine, Iowa State University.)

Figure 9.18. Parasympathetic Ganglion, Pulmonary Artery, Dog. A ganglion and associated nerve located in the adventitia of the artery.

Figure 9.19. Meissner's Plexus, Esophagus, x.s., Pig. These parasympathetic plexuses are located in the submucosa of the digestive tract. Note the characteristic large "owl's eye" nucleus of the neurons.

Figure 9.20. Auerbach's Plexus, Jejunum, l.s., Dog. These parasympathetic plexuses are located between the inner circular and outer longitudinal layers of the muscularis externa of the digestive tract.

Figure 9.21. Nerve, Myelinated, x.s., Pig (Masson's). The nerve shown is composed of many fascicles bounded by a connective tissue sheath, the epineurium. Each fascicle is surrounded by a perineurium and contains numerous axons.

Figure 9.19   × 125

Figure 9.20   × 62.5

Figure 9.22   × 260

KEY	
1. Axon	4. Perineurium
2. Endoneurium	5. Space artifact
3. Myelin sheath	

Figure 9.22. Nerve Fascicle (portion of), Myelinated, x.s., Pig (Masson's). Delicate connective tissue fibers of the endoneurium are visible around individual myelinated axons.

Figure 9.23   × 250

Figure 9.24   × 250

Figure 9.25   × 180

Figure 9.26   × 625

KEY	
1. Axon	5. Nerve fibers, l.s.
2. Blood vessel	6. Nerve fibers, x.s.
3. Groove in plasma membrane of Schwann cell	7. Perineurium
4. Myelin sheath	8. Schwann cell, nucleus

Figure 9.23. Nerve, Myelinated, Thoracic Wall, Cat. Myelin sheaths *(pink)* often present a scalloped or vacuolated appearance, an artifact of processing. Axons in this preparation are round, oval, or shriveled and either blue-gray or purple.

Figure 9.24. Axons, Myelinated, Medulla, Horse (Hagguist). Axons *(blue)* with myelin sheaths *(pink)* are seen in longitudinal sections and cross sections.

Figure 9.25. Nerve Fascicles, Unmyelinated, Ureter, Pig. Note the wavy appearance of the fibers that have been cut longitudinally. See Figure 9.26 for comment on relationship of axons to Schwann cells.

Figure 9.26. Nerve Fascicle (portion of), Unmyelinated, Left Ventricle, Pig. Each Schwann cell enwraps several unmyelinated axons within grooves (which appear as vesicles in cross section) of its plasma membrane. Axons can be seen filling some of the grooves, while in others they have shrunken from the plasma membrane of the Schwann cell.

Figure 9.27   × 25

Figure 9.31   × 12.5

Figure 9.28   × 62.5

KEY	
1. Arteriovenous shunt	9. Multipolar neurons
2. Capsule	10. Nerve
3. Central canal	11. Nuclear bag fiber
4. Fluid-filled space	12. Nuclear chain fiber
5. Glycogen body	13. Outer core
6. Gray matter	14. Pancreas
7. Inner core	15. Skeletal muscle, x.s.
8. Mesenteric blood vessel	16. White matter

Figure 9.27. Pacinian Corpuscle, whole mount, Mesentery, Cat (Carmine). Two corpuscles (one on the right somewhat distorted) are shown. Each is surrounded by a capsule of connective tissue within which are located concentric laminae of flattened cells that form the core. A nerve ending courses through the center of the corpuscle. The closely packed inner core cells surround the nerve. The peripheral laminae form a looser, outer core.

Figure 9.28. Pacinian Corpuscle, x.s., Pancreas, Cat. The pacinian corpuscle is frequently seen in the pancreas of carnivores. See Figure 9.27 for description.

Figure 9.29. Small Encapsulated Nerve Endings, Dermis, Planum, Cow. Numerous encapsulated sensory nerve endings occur in the dermis of the planum near the epithelium.

Figure 9.30. Neuromuscular Spindle, x.s., Thoracic Muscle, Cat. A neuromuscular spindle is a proprioceptor located within a muscle. It consists of sensory and motor nerve endings and intrafusal fibers, which are narrow, modified skeletal muscle cells. Nuclear chain fibers are intrafusal fibers with a single row of nuclei, while nuclear bag fibers are intrafusal fibers that contain many closely packed nuclei. A capsule encloses the fluid-filled space that surrounds the intrafusal fibers.

Figure 9.31. Glycogen Body, Lumbosacral Enlargement, Spinal Cord, x.s., Chicken. The glycogen body is found only in birds. It consists of polyhedral, vesicular cells, each containing a central mass of glycogen and a peripherally displaced nucleus.

Figure 9.29   × 125

Figure 9.30   × 250

Figure 9.32   × 62.5

Figure 9.33   × 12.5

Figure 9.34   × 62.5

Figure 9.36   × 62.5

KEY	
1. Axon	10. Muscle (moves feather)
2. Bone	11. Gray matter
3. Capsule of Herbst corpuscle	12. Multipolar neuron
4. Cell of glycogen body	13. Nerve
5. Central canal	14. Sharpey's fibers
6. Core	15. Space artifact
7. Dermis	16. Unipolar neuron
8. Dorsal root ganglion	17. Ventral root
9. Epidermis	18. White matter

Figure 9.32. Glycogen Body, Lumbosacral Enlargement, Spinal Cord, x.s., Chicken. Cells of the glycogen body in detail. See Figure 9.31 for description.

Figure 9.33. Dorsal Root Ganglion, Lumbosacral Enlargement, Spinal Cord, x.s., Chicken. Portions of the spinal cord, ventral root of a spinal nerve, dorsal root ganglion, and vertebra.

Figure 9.34. Dorsal Root Ganglion, Lumbosacral Enlargement, Spinal Cord, x.s., Chicken. Neuron cell bodies of unipolar neurons and myelinated axons are shown.

Figure 9.35. Herbst Corpuscle, Upper Beak, x.s., Chicken. These encapsulated nerve endings occur frequently in the skin of the bird. They are similar to pacinian corpuscles of mammals and consist of an outer capsule of connective tissue, a laminated core, and an axial sensory nerve ending.

Figure 9.36. Herbst Corpuscle, Skin, Neck, Chicken. The Herbst corpuscles associated with follicles of feathered skin are sausage-shaped.

Figure 9.35   × 125

10

CARDIOVASCULAR SYSTEM

The heart pumps blood and conveys it to the tissues and organs through blood vessels. Fluid that escapes from the blood is returned to the venous system by lymphatic vessels.

Vessels of the cardiovascular system are lined by an **endothelium,** which is, typically, a single layer of squamous cells. The smallest of the blood vessels, **capillaries,** are tiny endothelial tubes. They are easily overlooked in histologic sections, especially if they are compressed or collapsed.

The walls of arteries and veins are arranged into concentric layers: the inner **tunica intima,** middle **tunica media,** and outer **tunica adventitia.** The composition and thickness of these layers vary with the size and type of vessel. The tunica media is not always present.

Small arteries can be defined, arbitrarily, as possessing up to eight or nine layers of smooth muscle cells in the tunica media. The smallest of these vessels is usually termed an **arteriole.** Its wall is composed of an endothelium (tunica intima), one or two layers of circularly arranged smooth muscle cells (tunica media), and a bit of surrounding loose connective tissue (tunica adventitia). Some of the larger small arteries have an **internal elastic membrane.** Small arteries are accompanied by **small veins.** The smallest veins are called **venules.** These are similar to arterioles, but have relatively thin walls and lack a tunica media of smooth muscle. An internal elastic membrane is not found in small veins.

As the diameter of a vessel increases, the tunics become larger and more elaborate. For example, the tunica intima of a **medium artery** contains connective tissue interspersed between the endothelium and internal elastic membrane. The thick tunica media, with varying proportions of smooth muscle and elastic fibers, comprises the bulk of the wall. The connective tissue of the tunica adventitia contains collagenous and elastic fibers, small blood vessels (**vasa vasorum**), and nerves. A **medium vein,** in contrast, has less smooth muscle and fewer elastic fibers in the tunica media and possesses a thicker tunica adventitia.

Arteries ordinarily appear round in cross section and have an obvious, rippled, internal elastic membrane. Conversely, accompanying veins are larger in diameter with an irregular or collapsed lumen and thinner walls, and, except for some of the largest, they have no internal elastic membrane. The lumens of blood vessels in tissue sections often contain blood cells, plasma, or both. Although it can be difficult to distinguish between veins and **lymphatic vessels,** the latter have thinner walls than veins of similar size and normally do not contain erythrocytes. **Valves** may occur in both veins and lymphatic vessels.

There are several variations from the "typical" blood vessels: The tunica adventitia of large veins adjacent to the heart contains cardiac, rather than smooth, muscle. Some arteries have smooth muscle in the tunica intima, as well as the tunica media. Smooth muscle may be oriented either longitudinally or circularly. The tunica adventitia of arteries may be either abundant or scant.

The arteries of **arteriovenous anastomoses** lack an internal elastic membrane, but possess epithelioid (epithelial-like) longitudinally arranged smooth muscle cells. Special structures, the aortic and carotid bodies, are closely associated with the tunica adventitia of their respective arteries.

Many special vessels unique to certain organs such as the sinusoids of the liver, postcapillary venules of lymph nodes, and helicine arteries of the penis are presented elsewhere with their appropriate organ systems.

The **heart** is a muscular organ whose wall is composed of an **endocardium, myocardium,** and **epicardium.** The thickness and composition of the wall vary, being thickest in the ventricles and thinnest in the atria. The middle layer of cardiac muscle, the myocardium, predominates. Valves of connective tissue covered by an endothelium, are extensions of the endocardium. Regions of the heart, including the base of the aorta and pulmonary trunk, as well as the atrioventricular orifices and septum, are supported by the **cardiac skeleton.** This cardiac skeleton may be in the form of dense irregular connective tissue, fibrocartilage, hyaline cartilage, or bone and varies with age and among individuals.

A small amount of fluid occurs in the pericardial cavity between the epicardium (visceral pericardium) and the parietal pericardium.

Figure 10.1   × 250

Figure 10.2   × 625

Figure 10.3   × 125

Figure 10.4   × 250

Figure 10.5   × 250

KEY	
1. Arteriole, x.s.	9. Plasma cell
2. Capillary, l.s.	10. Skeletal muscle cell, x.s.
3. Capillary, x.s.	11. Small artery, x.s.
4. Endothelial cell, nucleus	12. Small vein
5. Endothelial cell, surface cut	13. Smooth muscle cell, nucleus
6. Erythrocytes	14. Uterine gland
7. Macrophage	15. Venule
8. Mast cell	

Figure 10.1. Capillaries, x.s. and l.s., Diaphragm, Dog. Extensive capillary networks occur around muscle cells.

Figure 10.2. Capillary, l.s., Lamina Propria, Duodenum, Sheep. Erythrocytes fill the lumen of this capillary.

Figure 10.3. Arterioles and Venules, Eyelid, Pig. Small blood vessels of various sizes are present in the dermis.

Figure 10.4. Arterioles, x.s., Endometrium, Uterus, Dog. The smallest of the arterioles shown have only one layer of smooth muscle in their walls.

Figure 10.5. Venule, l.s., Connective Tissue, Epiglottis, Goat. The wall of the venule consists of an endothelium surrounded by a small amount of connective tissue.

Figure 10.6   × 125

Figure 10.10   × 250

Figure 10.7   × 125

Figure 10.6. Arterioles and Venule, l.s., Submucosa, Esophagus, Cat. In the region where the arterioles have been cut tangentially, the circular arrangement of the smooth muscle of the tunica media can be seen.

Figure 10.7. Small Artery and Vein, x.s., Eyelid, Pig. These vessels are surrounded by portions of sweat glands in the dermis. Veins such as the one shown often have an irregular or collapsed lumen.

Figure 10.8. Small Artery, l.s., Esophagus, Pig.

Figure 10.9. Small Vein with Valve, l.s., Nose, Sheep. Valves are thin flaps of connective tissue covered on both sides by an endothelium.

Figure 10.10. Small Artery, x.s., with Branch, Subcutis, Dog.

Figure 10.8   × 125

Figure 10.9   × 125

Figure 10.11

× 62.5

Figure 10.15

× 62.5

Figure 10.12

× 125

Figure 10.13

× 62.5

Figure 10.14

× 62.5

KEY	
1. Adipose tissue	7. Nerve
2. Artery	8. Pancreas
3. Elastic fiber	9. Tunica adventitia
4. Erythrocytes	10. Tunica intima, endothelium
5. External elastic membrane	11. Tunica media
6. Internal elastic membrane	12. Vein

Figure 10.11. Small Artery, Vein, and Nerve, x.s., Pancreas, Cat. Note that both of the vessels have a sparse adventitia.

Figure 10.12. Artery and Vein, x.s., Wattle, Rooster. Note the especially thick tunica media of the artery.

Figure 10.13. Medium Artery, x.s., Lymph Node, Pig. The rich-pink color of the elastic fibers contrasts with the paler-pink color of the collagenous fibers and smooth muscle.

Figure 10.14. Medium Artery, x.s., Lymph Node, Pig (Orcein). Elastic fibers are stained reddish brown with orcein.

Figure 10.15. Medium Vein, l.s., Lymph Node, Pig. This vein accompanied the artery in Figures 10.13 and 10.14.

Figure 10.16   × 62.5

Figure 10.20   × 25

Figure 10.17   × 125

KEY	
1. Adipose tissue	5. Tunica adventitia
2. External elastic membrane	6. Tunica intima, endothelium
3. Internal elastic membrane	7. Tunica media
4. Nerve	8. Valve

Figure 10.16. Medium Vein, l.s., Lymph Node, Pig (Orcein). Elastic fibers are stained reddish brown with orcein.

Figure 10.17. Medium Artery, x.s., Lymph Node, Cat. Longitudinally oriented smooth muscle is present in the tunica intima between the endothelium and internal elastic membrane.

Figure 10.18. Renal Artery, Near Aorta, x.s., Pig. Note both an inner and outer layer of smooth muscle in the tunica media. The inner layer is arranged longitudinally.

Figure 10.19. Portal Vein, x.s., Dog. Note the bundles of longitudinally arranged smooth muscle in the tunica adventitia, a characteristic of large veins.

Figure 10.20. Vein with Valves, x.s., Lip, Pig.

Figure 10.18   × 62.5

Figure 10.19   × 62.5

Figure 10.21

× 12.5

Figure 10.25

× 12.5

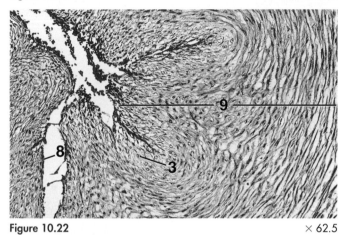

Figure 10.22

× 62.5

KEY	
1. Anastomotic artery	6. Tunica adventitia
2. Aorta, lumen	7. Tunica intima
3. Epithelioid cells	8. Tunica intima, endothelium
4. Nerve	9. Tunica media
5. Pulmonary artery, lumen	

Figure 10.21. Umbilical Artery (Right) and Vein (Left), x.s., Horse (Masson's). The tunica media of the umbilical artery is thicker than that of the umbilical vein.

Figure 10.22. Umbilical Artery, x.s., Horse (Masson's). The umbilical artery lacks an internal elastic membrane. The innermost smooth muscle cells of the tunica media are epithelioid (epithelial-like) and oriented longitudinally.

Figure 10.23. Glomus, Nose, Pig. The highly convoluted anastomotic artery, surrounding connective tissue, and nerves forming this organized arteriovenous anastomosis can be seen.

Figure 10.24. Arteriovenous Anastomosis, x.s., Lip, Pig. Longitudinally directed cells of smooth muscle of the tunica media are characteristically epithelioid (epithelial-like) in an anastomotic artery. These arteries lack an internal elastic membrane and have a small lumen.

Figure 10.25. Aorta (Left) and Pulmonary Artery (Right), x.s., Pig (Orcein). This preparation was stained with orcein to highlight elastic tissue *(red-brown).*

Figure 10.23

× 125

Figure 10.24

× 250

Figure 10.26   × 62.5

Figure 10.30   × 25

Figure 10.27   × 62.5

KEY	
1. Adipose tissue	6. Myocardium
2. Cardiac muscle	7. Smooth muscle
3. Collagenous fibers	8. Tunica intima, endothelium
4. Elastic fibers	9. Tunica media
5. Endocardium	10. Vasa vasorum

Figure 10.26. Aorta, x.s., Dog (Orcein). This specimen was stained with orcein to emphasize elastic tissue *(red-brown).*

Figure 10.27. Pulmonary Artery, x.s., Sheep. Portion of the tunica intima and tunica media. Smooth muscle of the tunica media is oriented in various directions. Wavy, pink elastic fibers occur among the smooth muscle.

Figure 10.28. Vena Cava, x.s., Dog. This section was taken from a region near the heart. The tunica adventitia consists largely of cardiac muscle and adipose tissue.

Figure 10.29. Right Auricle, Pig (Orcein). The section was stained with orcein to show the distribution of elastic fibers *(red-brown).*

Figure 10.30. Right Auricle, Pig (Mallory's). This preparation shows the distribution of smooth muscle in the endocardium.

Figure 10.28   × 62.5

Figure 10.29   × 25

Figure 10.31   × 12.5

Figure 10.31. Pulmonic (Semilunar) Valve, x.s., Dog. Pulmonic valves are located in the pulmonary artery near the heart. The section shows a portion of the fibrous cardiac skeleton.

Figure 10.32. Pulmonic (Semilunar) Valve, x.s., Dog (Masson's). Portions of two adjacent pulmonic valves are visible. The connective tissue of the valves and the tunica media of the pulmonary artery blend with the fibrous cardiac skeleton. A cushion of mesenchyme-like connective tissue lies adjacent to the cardiac skeleton.

Figure 10.33. Pulmonic (Semilunar) Valve, x.s., Dog. The valve consists of a core of dense irregular connective tissue sandwiched between two layers of endothelium.

Figure 10.34. Pulmonic (Semilunar) Valve, x.s., Dog. A portion of the atrial wall, pulmonary artery, aorta, and cardiac skeleton (cartilaginous and fibrous) are visible.

Figure 10.32   × 25

Figure 10.33   × 62.5

Figure 10.34   × 12.5

Figure 10.35 × 125

Figure 10.37 × 62.5

Figure 10.36 × 180

Figure 10.38 × 125

KEY		
1. Adipose tissue		8. Parenchyma cells
2. Arteriole		9. Pericardial cavity
3. Chondrocyte		10. Pericardium, parietal
4. Myocardium, right ventricle		11. Pericardium, visceral
5. Myofibrils		12. Purkinje cell, l.s.
6. Nerve		13. Purkinje cell, x.s.
7. Neuron cell body		

Figure 10.35. Cardiac Skeleton, Dog. The cartilaginous portion of the cardiac skeleton of the dog is formed from fibrocartilage containing numerous scattered chondrocytes.

Figure 10.36. Purkinje Cells, x.s. and l.s., Left Ventricle, Goat. Myofibrils are limited to the periphery of these large, modified cardiac muscle cells.

Figure 10.37. Visceral and Parietal Pericardium, Cat. The pericardium consists of a mesothelium (simple squamous epithelium) and underlying connective tissue. The mesothelium of the visceral pericardium (epicardium) covers the surface of the heart. The remainder of the pericardial cavity is lined by the mesothelium of the parietal pericardium.

Figure 10.38. Aortic Body, Pig. The aortic body is located between the pulmonary artery and aorta. It is a small, encapsulated structure containing blood vessels, nerves, and two types of parenchyma cells (see Fig. 10.39).

Figure 10.39

× 250

Figure 10.39. Aortic Body, Pig. Two types of parenchyma cells can be distinguished in the aortic body. The type I (glomus) cell has a round nucleus and a granular cytoplasm. The type II (sustentacular) cell has few or no cytoplasmic granules and an oval nucleus. Type I cells usually occur in clusters surrounded by Type II cells and connective tissue.

Figure 10.40. Lymphatic Vessel with Valve, Artery, and Vein, Cecal Tonsil, Chicken. Lymphatic vessels have a large lumen and a relatively thin wall. Valves may be present.

Figure 10.41. Lymphatic Vessel with Valve, Lymph Node, Pig. The valves of lymphatic vessels consist of a connective tissue core surrounded on each side by an endothelium.

Figure 10.42. Large Lymphatic Vessel, Submucosa, Cecum, Horse. The wall of the lymphatic vessel consists of an endothelium surrounded by a small amount of connective tissue. The latter blends with the connective tissue of the submucosa.

Figure 10.40

× 62.5

Figure 10.41

× 62.5

Figure 10.42

× 62.5

11

LYMPHATIC SYSTEM

Lymphatic tissue consists predominantly of lymphocytes. These and a variable number of plasma cells, macrophages, and other cells occur among a framework of reticular cells and fibers. In H&E preparations lymphatic tissue appears purple because of the presence of numerous small lymphocytes, each with a basophilic nucleus and little cytoplasm.

MAMMALS

Diffuse lymphatic tissue is characterized by a moderate concentration of scattered lymphocytes. A round, oval, or irregularly circumscribed aggregation of mostly small, densely packed lymphocytes is called a **lymphatic nodule**. A nodule may contain a central pale area, the **germinal center**. Because the majority of cells of the germinal center are larger lymphocytes with more cytoplasm and lightly staining nuclei, this region appears pale in contrast to the dense **corona** (marginal zone, peripheral zone) of small lymphocytes. Diffuse lymphatic tissue and lymphatic nodules are components of most lymphatic organs. They also appear in the connective tissue of the digestive, respiratory, urinary, and reproductive organs, among other locations.

Aggregations of lymphatic nodules form **Peyer's patches** in the lamina propria and submucosa of the small intestine, particularly the ileum.

Tonsils are collections of lymphatic nodules and diffuse lymphatic tissue. They occur in the connective tissue below the epithelium in specific regions of the tongue, pharynx, and larynx.

Follicular tonsils are characterized by deep invaginations of the surface epithelium called crypts. A crypt together with its associated lymphatic tissue is a **tonsillar follicle**. Collectively, several follicles form the tonsil. Examples of tonsils with crypts include the following: **lingual tonsils** of the horse, pig, and cow; **tubal tonsils** of the pig; **paraepiglottic tonsils** of the pig, sheep, and goat; **palatine tonsils** of the horse, pig, and ruminant. In the palatine tonsils of ruminants the crypts lead into a common sinus, which then opens onto the surface.

Tonsils without crypts have a smooth, somewhat folded, or bulging surface, but lack deep invaginations of the epithelium. Examples of these are the **tubal tonsils** of ruminants, the **paraepiglottic tonsil** of the cat, and the **palatine tonsils** of carnivores.

Salivary glands associated with tonsils are typically mucous glands except those in carnivores, where they are mixed (mucous and serous combined).

A **lymph node** is organized into a cortex and medulla. The cortex consists of lymphatic nodules surrounded by diffuse lymphatic tissue. Extensions of the latter tissue into the medulla are called medullary cords. Lymphocytes, other leukocytes, macrophages, and plasma cells can be found in the medullary cords.

A **capsule** of connective tissue, with some smooth muscle and elastic fibers, covers the lymph node. Parts of the capsule extend inward as **trabeculae.** Afferent lymphatic vessels penetrate the capsule to join the subcapsular sinus. Cortical sinuses connect the **subcapsular sinus** to **medullary sinuses.** The latter lead to efferent lymphatic vessels at the hilus. The various sinuses are less cellular than the parenchyma and appear pale by comparison. They are lined by a discontinuous endothelium and are spanned by a webwork of cytoplasmic processes of reticular cells. They contain some free cells such as lymphocytes and macrophages.

Blood vessels enter and leave the node mostly from the region of the hilus. Unique blood vessels called **postcapillary venules** are found in the deep cortex. They are lined by elongated cells that appear cuboidal when cut in cross section. Lymphocytes migrate between these cells.

The amount or arrangement of cortical and medullary tissue can vary from that of the "typical" lymph node. The lymph node of the pig, for example, is characteristically atypical with the location of the cortical and medullary tissue, as well as the flow of lymph, being reversed.

Hemal nodes occur along blood vessels of ruminants. They are characterized by blood-filled sinuses between cellular cords. Connective tissue and some smooth muscle form the capsule and trabeculae (which are sparse). Hemal nodes lack lymphatic vessels. **Hemolymph nodes,** in contrast to hemal nodes, possess lymphatic vessels. Their sinuses receive a mixture of blood and lymph.

The **spleen** has a **capsule** that is rich in smooth muscle and elastic fibers. In horses and cows two or three layers of muscle are oriented perpendicular to each other, while in carnivores, pigs, sheep, and goats the muscle fibers are interwoven. The capsule is thickest in the horse and cow and thinnest in carnivores. **Trabeculae** project into the interior of the spleen from the capsule. They tend to be especially large in cows and sheep.

The parenchyma of the spleen is divisible into the white and red pulp. Dense accumulations of lymphocytes, arranged around central arteries, form the **periarterial lymphatic sheaths** (PALS). These, along with lymphatic nodules, comprise the **white pulp.** White pulp appears purple in H&E preparations because of the high concentration of numerous small lymphocytes. **Red pulp,** because of the large numbers of erythrocytes it contains in its reticular meshwork and blood vessels, is stained red in H&E preparations.

The **splenic artery** enters the hilus of the spleen and branches into **trabecular arteries.** When these enter the parenchyma of the spleen and become surrounded by white pulp, they are called **central arteries** (not necessarily located in the center of the PALS). On leaving the white pulp, the central artery branches into a group of **pulp arteries.** These, in turn, branch into two or three **arterioles,** which terminate in two or more **capillaries.** Commonly, the pulp arteries and their branches are called a **penicillus** because, collectively, they resemble the bristles of an artist's brush. A portion of the capillaries of the penicillus becomes surrounded by concentric layers of macrophages contained in a reticular framework. These cellular and fibrous thickenings are called **ellipsoids** (pericapillary macrophage sheaths). The term **sheathed capillary** is used by some authors for the combined unit consisting of the capillary and the ellipsoid. Ellipsoids are especially abundant in the **marginal zone,** the region between the red and white pulp. They are very large and numerous in pigs. The capillaries of the ellipsoids continue as terminal arterial capillaries. Arterial capillaries may join venous sinuses or pulp veins (closed circulation), or they may empty directly into the spaces of the reticular meshwork of the red pulp (open circulation).

The spleen of the dog is a **sinusal** spleen. The red pulp contains typical **venous** (splenic, vascular) **sinuses.** These are wide channels lined by elongated, longitudinally oriented endothelial cells. The spleens of the cat, horse, pig, and ruminant are classified as **nonsinusal,** having poorly developed or no sinuses. Wisps of smooth muscle in the red pulp are most numerous in pigs and ruminants.

The **thymus** gland is covered by a thin capsule of connective tissue that projects inward as **septa,** partially dividing the organ into **lobules.** The parenchyma of each lobule is organized into a **cortex** of mostly small, densely packed lymphocytes and a **medulla** with fewer and larger lymphocytes. The medulla is continuous between lobules. The thymus lacks lymphatic nodules and is supported by a unique cytoreticulum of stellate, epithelial reticular cells and only a few reticular fibers.

Hassall's (thymic) **corpuscles** occur in the medulla of each lobule. They are concentric whorls of acidophilic and flattened reticular cells that may become swollen, keratinized, and calcified centrally. They are found exclusively in the thymus gland.

As an animal ages, much of the thymus becomes replaced by adipose tissue.

CHICKEN

Lymph nodes do not occur in the chicken. However, diffuse lymphatic tissue and lymphatic nodules are widespread.

The **spleen** of the chicken is covered by a muscular capsule, but trabeculae are absent. Areas of red and white pulp are less distinct than in the mammalian spleen. **White pulp** is diffusely scattered throughout the spleen and is composed primarily of small lymphocytes. It contains **sheathed arteries** and, occasionally, lymphatic nodules. **Red pulp** is formed from venous sinuses and anastomosing cords of reticular cells, macrophages, lymphocytes, and red blood cells.

As in mammals, the **thymus** is arranged into incompletely separated lobules of cortical and medullary tissue. Typical Hassall's corpuscles, similar to those found in mammals, are seen infrequently. Instead, diffuse forms of Hassall's corpuscles, called **reticular structures,** are abundant in the medulla. These are pale, irregular masses of reticular cells with vesicles that contain acidophilic material and degenerating cells. **Myoid cells,** characterized by a fibrous cytoplasm, also occur in the medulla.

The **bursa of Fabricius** is a saclike dorsal diverticulum of the proctodeum that is unique to birds. It is characterized by tall, thick mucosal **folds** (plicae) filled with numerous polyhedral **follicles.** Each follicle, composed of lymphatic tissue, is divided into a **cortex** and **medulla.** A layer of **undifferentiated epithelial cells** occupies the periphery of the medulla, which is separated from the cortex by a **capillary layer.** The bursa is lined by a pseudostratified columnar epithelium, except at the apex of each follicle, which is covered by an **epithelial tuft** of simple columnar cells.

Figure 11.1 ×25

Figure 11.2 ×12.5

Figure 11.3 ×250

Figure 11.4 ×250

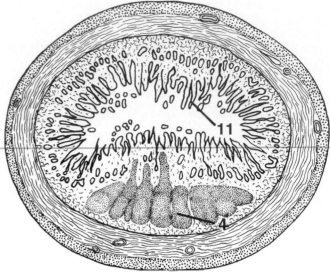

Figure 11.5

KEY	
1. Corona	7. Mucosa
2. Diffuse lymphatic tissue	8. Muscularis externa
3. Germinal center	9. Reticular cell
4. Lymphatic nodule	10. Submucosa
5. Lymphocyte, large	11. Villus
6. Lymphocyte, small	

Figure 11.1. Lymphatic Nodules and Diffuse Lymphatic Tissue, Pyloric Stomach, Cat. Dense aggregations of lymphocytes form lymphatic nodules in the lamina propria.

Figure 11.2. Lymphatic Nodules and Diffuse Lymphatic Tissue, Colon, x.s., Pig. The mucosa and submucosa contain diffuse lymphatic tissue and large lymphatic nodules with germinal centers. Lymphatic nodules are especially numerous in the digestive tract of the pig.

Figure 11.3. Lymphatic Nodule, Colon, Pig. Cells of the germinal center and corona. Many small lymphocytes occur in the peripheral corona; fewer and larger cells are seen in the germinal center.

Figure 11.4. Lymphatic Nodule, Colon, Pig. Detail of cells of the germinal center and corona. Small lymphocytes are characterized by a heterochromatic nucleus and scant cytoplasm.

Figure 11.5. Peyer's Patch, Ileum, x.s., Cat. A Peyer's patch is an aggregation of lymphatic nodules in the lamina propria and submucosa of the small intestine.

Figure 11.6 ×12.5

Figure 11.7 ×12.5

Figure 11.8

Figure 11.9 ×12.5

Figure 11.10 ×125

KEY	
1. Diffuse lymphatic tissue	10. Skeletal muscle
2. Epiglottis	11. Stratified squamous epithelium, semilunar fold
3. Fossa	
4. Lymphatic nodule	12. Stratified squamous epithelium, tonsil
5. Mucous acinus	
6. Muscularis externa	13. Submucosa
7. Salivary glands	14. Vestibular fold
8. Serous acinus	15. Villus
9. Serous demilune	

Figure 11.6. Peyer's Patch, Ileum, x.s., Dog. Eight lymphatic nodules of a portion of a Peyer's patch are visible in this section.

Figure 11.7. Paraepiglottic Tonsil, Larynx, l.s., Cat. In the cat an accumulation of lymphatic tissue in the lateral wall of the larynx, between the epiglottis and the vestibular fold, forms a tonsil without crypts.

Figure 11.8. Palatine Tonsil, Dog. In the dog the entire tonsil lies within a fossa (a small hollow) and is covered in part by a semilunar fold. The palatine tonsils of carnivores lack crypts.

Figure 11.9. Palatine Tonsil, Dog. A portion of a tonsil and semilunar fold.

Figure 11.10. Palatine Tonsil, Dog. Mixed salivary glands are associated with the wall of the tonsils in carnivores. In other species only mucous glands are present.

Figure 11.11

Figure 11.15   ×12.5

Figure 11.12   ×12.5

KEY	
1. Capsule	8. Medullary cord
2. Cortical sinus	9. Medullary sinus
3. Crypt	10. Salivary glands, mucous
4. Deep cortex	11. Stratified squamous epithelium
5. Diffuse lymphatic tissue	12. Subcapsular sinus
6. Leukocyte infiltration	13. Trabecula
7. Lymphatic nodule	

Figure 11.11. Palatine Tonsil, Horse. The palatine tonsils of non-carnivores have crypts (surface invaginations lined by stratified squamous epithelium).

Figure 11.12. Palatine Tonsil, Horse. Note that the continuity of each crypt with the surface is not always evident.

Figure 11.13. Palatine Tonsil, Horse. Lymphocytes and other leukocytes have infiltrated and partly obliterated the epithelial lining of this crypt.

Figure 11.14. Lymph Node, Cow. The lymph node is surrounded by a capsule. Trabeculae project inward from the capsule. The cortex contains sinuses, diffuse lymphatic tissue, and lymphatic nodules. The medulla is composed of medullary cords and sinuses.

Figure 11.15. Lymph Node, Dog.

Figure 11.13   ×125

Figure 11.14

Figure 11.16 ×12.5

Figure 11.17 ×12.5

Figure 11.18 ×12.5

Figure 11.19 ×12.5

Figure 11.20 ×12.5

KEY	
1. Capsule	6. Lymphatic nodule
2. Cartilage plate, bronchus	7. Medulla, lymph node
3. Cortex, lymph node	8. Medullary cord
4. Cortical tissue	9. Medullary sinus
5. Diffuse lymphatic tissue	10. Primary bronchus, lumen

Figure 11.16. Tracheobronchial Lymph Node, Dog. This lymph node is adjacent to the wall of a primary bronchus near the tracheal bifurcation.

Figure 11.17. Lymph Node, Horse. The arrangement of cortical and medullary tissues may be atypical in some of the lymph nodes of mammals. In the example shown the distribution of cortical and medullary components is the reverse of that commonly expected.

Figure 11.18. Lymph Node, Horse. Not only is the arrangement of cortical and medullary components reversed in this section, but the proportion of the medullary tissue is much greater than usual.

Figure 11.19. Lymph Node, Pig. The lymph nodes of pigs consistently show an atypical pattern. In this section cortical tissue is predominantly central, while medullary tissue occurs both superficially and internally.

Figure 11.20. Lymph Node, Cow. The lymph node of the cow is often characterized by the presence of large lymphatic nodules.

Figure 11.21 ×62.5

Figure 11.25 ×125

Figure 11.22 ×125

KEY	
1. Capsule	5. Reticular fiber
2. Cortical sinus	6. Smooth muscle
3. Diffuse lymphatic tissue	7. Subcapsular sinus
4. Lymphatic nodule	8. Trabecula

Figure 11.21. Cortex, Lymph Node, Horse. The subcapsular sinus below the capsule continues as cortical sinuses that parallel the trabeculae through the cortex.

Figure 11.22. Cortex, Lymph Node, Cow (Masson's). The inner portion of the capsule contains smooth muscle *(pink).*

Figure 11.23. Cortex, Lymph Node, Cow. The trabecula contains smooth muscle.

Figure 11.24. Cortex, Lymph Node, Cow (Silver). A network of fine, branching reticular fibers provides a supportive framework for the diffuse and nodular lymphatic tissue.

Figure 11.25. Cortex, Lymph Node, Sheep (Mallory's). Continuity of the subcapsular sinus with the cortical sinus is evident.

Figure 11.23 ×125

Figure 11.24 ×125

Figure 11.26 ×250

Figure 11.30 ×125

Figure 11.27 ×250

Figure 11.26. Cortex, Lymph Node, Sheep (Mallory's). Smooth muscle cells *(pink)* among collagenous fibers *(blue)* of the capsule.

Figure 11.27. Deep Cortex, Lymph Node, Dog. Postcapillary venules, l.s. and x.s. These vessels are lined by elongated cells that appear cuboidal in cross section. Lymphocytes migrate between the endothelial cells of the postcapillary venules.

Figure 11.28. Cortex, Lymph Node, Horse. Multinucleate giant cells, derived from the coalescence of macrophages, are sometimes found in lymph nodes.

Figure 11.29. Medulla, Lymph Node, Cow. In this preparation reticular cells, endothelial cells, and macrophages contain numerous pigment granules.

Figure 11.30. Medulla, Lymph Node, Sheep. Smooth muscle is distributed throughout the medullary sinuses.

Figure 11.28 ×125

Figure 11.29 ×250

Figure 11.31

×250

Figure 11.34

×250

Figure 11.31. Medulla, Lymph Node, Dog. Cellular medullary cords surround medullary sinuses that are lined incompletely by endothelial cells. A megakaryocyte is present in a medullary cord.

Figure 11.32. Medulla, Lymph Node, Dog. Macrophages containing phagocytized erythrocytes are evident in the medullary sinuses.

Figure 11.33. Hemal Node, Sheep. The general organization is much like that of a lymph node, but the sinuses are filled with blood. Lymphatic nodules are scarce, and trabeculae of connective tissue are not apparent.

Figure 11.34. Hemal Node, Sheep. The subcapsular (marginal) sinus is filled with blood. Reticular cells of the sinus contain phagocytized material.

Figure 11.32

×360

Figure 11.33

×25

Figure 11.35

Figure 11.39   ×62.5

Figure 11.36   ×12.5

KEY	
1. Capsule	7. Mesothelium
2. Central artery	8. Red pulp
3. Ellipsoid	9. Trabecula
4. Endothelial cell	10. Venous sinus
5. Lymphatic nodule	11. White pulp
6. Marginal zone	

Figure 11.35. Spleen, Dog. This drawing is of a small portion of the spleen.

Figure 11.36. Spleen, Dog. The parenchyma of the spleen is organized into red pulp and white pulp (periarterial lymphatic sheaths and lymphatic nodules). Trabeculae extend inward from the capsule and are seen throughout the red pulp.

Figure 11.37. Spleen, Dog. Note the smooth muscle in the capsule and trabeculae. The spleen of the dog is a sinusal spleen, containing venous sinuses (see Fig. 11.38).

Figure 11.38. Spleen, Dog. Venous sinuses are lined by longitudinally oriented, elongated endothelial cells. The nuclei may or may not be apparent in cross sections of such lining cells. Erythrocytes fill the sinuses and the spaces of the red pulp.

Figure 11.39. Spleen, Dog. Ellipsoids can be seen in the marginal zone between the periarterial lymphatic sheath (white pulp) and the red pulp. They are also present in the red pulp.

Figure 11.37   ×62.5

Figure 11.38   ×250

Figure 11.40   ×125

Figure 11.41   ×25

Figure 11.42   ×62.5

Figure 11.43   ×62.5

Figure 11.44   ×62.5

KEY	
1. Capillary lumen	7. Periarterial lymphatic sheath
2. Capsule	8. Red pulp
3. Central Artery	9. Serosa
4. Elastic fiber	10. Smooth muscle
5. Ellipsoid	11. Trabecula
6. Marginal zone	

Figure 11.40. Spleen, Pig (Orcein). The capsule and trabeculae are rich in elastic fibers *(red-brown).*

Figure 11.41. Spleen, Pig (Mallory's). Ellipsoids are abundant in the pig. They are especially numerous in the vicinity of the marginal zone of a periarterial lymphatic sheath. See Figure 11.44 for details of ellipsoids.

Figure 11.42. Capsule, Spleen, Horse. The capsule of the spleen of the horse and cow contains layers of smooth muscle oriented at right angles to each other, rather than being interwoven as in carnivores, pigs, sheep, and goats. In this preparation there are three distinct layers of muscle. Compare with Figures 11.37, 11.43, and 11.45.

Figure 11.43. Capsule, Spleen, Cow. The capsule contains two thick layers of smooth muscle oriented at right angles to each other.

Figure 11.44. Spleen, Pig. Ellipsoids are especially abundant in the spleen of the pig. Each consists of macrophages and reticular fibers that surround a capillary.

Figure 11.45   ×62.5

Figure 11.46   ×25

Figure 11.47   ×125

Figure 11.48   ×12.5

Figure 11.45. Capsule, Spleen, Sheep. In sheep the bulk of the capsule contains many interwoven smooth muscle cells. The smooth muscle in the capsule of the spleen of carnivores (see Fig. 11.37), pigs, and goats has a similar arrangement. In the horse (see Fig. 11.42) and cow (see Fig. 11.43) the muscle cells are arranged in layers instead. Elastic fibers can be observed as faint pink spirals.

Figure 11.46. Spleen, Sheep. Note the thick trabecula. Characteristically, the spleens of cows and sheep have thick trabeculae. Compare with Figure 11.41.

Figure 11.47. Red Pulp, Spleen, Sheep. Wisps of smooth muscle are scattered throughout the red pulp.

Figure 11.48. Thymus, Puppy. A thin capsule of connective tissue covers the thymus. Lobules, incompletely divided by connective-tissue septa, consist of an outer, dark cortex and an inner, pale medulla. The medulla is continuous between adjacent lobules.

Figure 11.49

×260

KEY		
1. Cortex		3. Medulla
2. Hassall's corpuscle		

Figure 11.49. Thymus, Puppy. Portion of the medulla and cortex. The cortex consists predominantly of small lymphocytes. The lymphocytes of the medulla are larger and less abundant. The medulla contains concentrically arranged, swollen, and keratinized reticular cells that form Hassall's corpuscles, which are characteristic of the thymus.

Figure 11.50   ×12.5

Figure 11.51   ×12.5

Figure 11.52   ×25

Figure 11.53   ×250

Figure 11.54   ×360

Figure 11.50. Thymus, Cat (old). In older animals functional thymic tissue is largely supplanted by adipose tissue.

Figure 11.51. Cecal Tonsil, x.s., Chicken. The accumulation of diffuse and nodular lymphatic tissue in the lamina propria and submucosa near the opening of each cecum is called the cecal tonsil.

Figure 11.52. Spleen, Chicken. Red pulp *(pink)* intermingles with white pulp *(purple)*. The white pulp contains a few lymphatic nodules. Trabeculae of connective tissue are absent.

Figure 11.53. Capsule, Spleen, Chicken. Layers of smooth muscle make up a substantial part of the capsule.

Figure 11.54. Spleen, Chicken. Sheathed arteries, x.s., in white pulp. These vessels are lined by plump endothelial cells surrounded by reticular cells.

Figure 11.55 ×12.5

Figure 11.59 ×250

Figure 11.56 ×250

KEY	
1. Bursa of Fabricius, lumen	8. Muscularis
2. Capillary layer	9. Myoid cell
3. Cortex	10. Pseudostratified epithelium
4. Epithelial tuft	11. Reticular structure
5. Follicle	12. Septum
6. Lamina propria	13. Undifferentiated epithelial cell
7. Medulla	14. Vesicle

Figure 11.55. Thymus, Chicken. The thymus of the chicken is similar to that of mammals. The pale areas throughout the medullary regions of the lobules are called reticular structures (see Fig. 11.56).

Figure 11.56. Medulla, Thymus, Chicken. Myoid cells, cut obliquely, are characterized by a fibrous cytoplasm and peripheral nuclei. The pale-staining reticular structure in this section is considered a diffuse form of a Hassall's corpuscle. It consists of diffuse groups of reticular cells and scattered vesicles. The vesicles may contain eosinophilic material or degenerating cells.

Figure 11.57. Bursa of Fabricius, Chicken. Portions of the long mucosal folds (plicae) project into the lumen of the bursa. Numerous follicles, each composed of a cortex and medulla, fill the lamina propria of each fold.

Figure 11.58. Bursa of Fabricius, Chicken. Where the apex of a follicle contacts the epithelium, tall, pale columnar cells with apical nuclei form an epithelial tuft. Elsewhere, mucosal folds are covered by a pseudostratified columnar epithelium.

Figure 11.59. Bursa of Fabricius, Chicken. A portion of a follicle. The darkly stained cortex is composed mostly of many small lymphocytes. The paler medulla contains fewer cells of various sizes. A layer of undifferentiated epithelial cells, which are cuboidal with an acidophilic cytoplasm, occupies the periphery of the medulla. A capillary network separates the cortex and the medulla.

Figure 11.57 ×12.5

Figure 11.58 ×125

12

INTEGUMENT

The integument includes the skin and its derivatives. Skin consists of an epidermis and dermis joined to underlying structures such as muscle and bone by the subcutis (subcutaneous tissue). Sweat, sebaceous, and mammary glands, as well as hair and feather follicles, are epidermal structures that are located in the dermis and subcutis. The highly keratinized claws and hooves of mammals and the beak, claws, and scales of fowl are also skin derivatives.

MAMMALS

The **epidermis** of **thick skin** is a keratinized, stratified, squamous epithelium. The **stratum basale** is a single layer of cuboidal to columnar cells that lies on a basement membrane adjacent to the dermis. These cells give rise to the **stratum spinosum,** a layer of variable thickness, whose polygonal cells become squamous toward the surface. Cells of the **stratum granulosum** contain basophilic keratohyalin granules in their cytoplasm. The **stratum lucidum** is a thin, pale, eosinophilic, translucent layer. It is limited to regions where the epidermis is very thick such as the digital pads of carnivores. In structures composed of hard keratin (rather than soft keratin) such as hooves and claws, both the stratum granulosum and stratum lucidum are absent. The most superficial layer of skin, the **stratum corneum,** is composed of dead, keratinized squamous cells that slough from the surface. Cell division within the stratum basale and stratum spinosum allows continued growth of the epidermis.

The epidermis of **thin skin** is composed of relatively few cells, but the number varies with the location. Thin skin lacks a stratum lucidum, and a stratum granulosum is not always evident.

The **dermis** consists of loose and dense irregular connective tissue containing blood vessels, lymphatic vessels, and nerves. In thick skin the superficial, loose connective tissue of the dermis, the **papillary layer**, forms projections called **dermal papillae** that interdigitate with the epidermis and serve to anchor the two layers. The deep layer of dense irregular connective tissue of thick skin is called the **reticular layer**.

In thin skin dermal papillae are either reduced or absent. Therefore, when both loose and dense irregular connective-tissue layers can be distinguished in the dermis of thin skin, they are best referred to as the superficial and deep layers, respectively.

Hairs are associated with regions of the body covered by thin skin. They arise from **germinal** (matrix) **cells** of the **hair bulb** at the base of the follicle. Multiplication of germinal cells results in growth of the hair. Near its origin, a hair consists of a central **medulla** of cuboidal cells, a **cortex** of flattened cells oriented parallel to the long axis of the hair, and an outer **cuticle** consisting of scalelike cells that partially overlap so their free edges are directed upward toward the surface of the skin. As the cells of the hair are pushed toward the surface from the region of the hair bulb, they become keratinized. Within the hair the medulla may become reduced distally, and it is absent entirely in wool hairs.

Hair follicles are set obliquely in the dermis or subcutis, although in sheep they tend to be vertical. A vascular **dermal papilla** projects into the hair bulb. **Melanocytes,** located close to the dermal papilla among matrix cells, have cytoplasmic processes that provide pigment to the hair cells. The germinal cells of the matrix, in addition to forming new hair cells, give rise to the **inner root sheath** of the follicle. The **cuticle of the inner root sheath** is composed of overlapping, scalelike cells similar to those of the cuticle of the hair, but their free edges are directed downward, so that the hair and inner-root sheath interlock. The inner root sheath becomes keratinized and tapers distally, ending close to the opening of sebaceous glands into the follicle. The peripheral **external root sheath** represents a downward continuation of the epidermis. A connective tissue (dermal) **sheath** surrounds the follicle and abuts the **basement** (glassy) **membrane** of the external root sheath. It blends with the rest of the dermal connective tissue. An **arrector pili muscle** (smooth muscle) inserts on the connective tissue sheath of the follicle and originates from the superficial layer of the dermis.

Single (simple) **hair follicles** are evenly distributed in the skin of horses and ruminants and occur in groups of three in pigs. In carnivores most of the follicles are **compound follicles**. Each compound follicle is formed from a single primary follicle and several secondary follicles. The follicles unite at the level of the openings of the sebaceous glands, forming a common follicle, which extends from the point of union to the skin surface. The hairs that are produced exit as a group to the surface through the common follicular opening. **Sinus** (tactile) **hairs** are limited to the face region. They are produced by large follicles that are well innervated and that contain blood-filled sinuses within their connective-tissue sheaths. In horses, pigs, and ruminants the sinus is trabeculated throughout its length. In carnivores the upper region is nontrabeculated, forming an annular sinus.

The short ducts of **sebaceous glands** usually empty into hair follicles, although they may also empty directly onto the skin surface. Basal (stem) cells of sebaceous glands divide and give rise to vacuolated secretory cells that synthesize lipid. The innermost, mature secretory cells die and break apart, forming an oily product called sebum. This form of product release is called holocrine secretion.

Sweat glands may be winding (serpentine) or highly coiled and may be either tubular or saclike. They empty their secretion through a duct, either into a hair follicle or onto the skin surface. The epithelium of the secretory portion of the gland varies from flattened to columnar. Contractile **myoepithelial cells** surround the secretory cells and the initial portion of their ducts.

Traditionally, sweat glands have been classified as either merocrine (secretory product released by exocytosis) or apocrine (secretory product released when small pieces of cytoplasm containing the product are pinched off the free surface of the cell). Recent evidence, however, has suggested that this may not be true and that all sweat glands may use the merocrine form of release. We have chosen to use the traditional nomenclature until the matter is resolved.

Special regions in the skin of various species have numerous, well-developed glands. The carpal glands of pigs consist of masses of merocrine sweat glands. Numerous apocrine sweat glands characterize the mental organ of pigs and the interdigital and inguinal pouches of sheep. The submental organ of cats, the supracaudal gland of carnivores, the infraorbital pouch of sheep, and the scent (horn) glands of goats contain many large sebaceous glands.

The skin of the **nose** of horses is thin with fine hairs, sebaceous and sweat glands, and occasional sinus hairs. The planum of the nose of the other domestic mammals is covered by a thick, highly keratinized epidermis. The planum nasale of carnivores is devoid of glands and hairs. In cats the epidermis forms numerous small bumps, while that of the dog is rather flat with surface grooves. The planum rostrale of the pig contains numerous merocrine sweat glands and sparse hairs. The planum nasolabiale of the cow and the planum nasale of sheep and goats are hairless and contain compound acinar glands that produce a serous secretion.

Digital pads of cats and dogs are covered by a very thick epidermis that is smooth in the dog and roughened by conical papillae in the cat. Coiled merocrine sweat glands occur in the dermis and the digital cushion of the pads.

Lobules of **mammary glands** are situated in the subcutis and consist of tubuloacinar glands and intralobular ducts. When a mammary gland is active, secretory tissue is prominent, and intralobular and interlobular connective tissue is reduced. When a gland is inactive, only the duct system is evident. Cellular thickenings at the termination of intralobular ducts represent gland remnants or gland precursors in the inactive gland. Interlobular ducts, with a bistratified cuboidal to columnar lining, drain the lobules and lead to the lactiferous ducts and lactiferous sinuses at the base of the teat. The teat sinus, with a bistratified columnar to cuboidal lining, leads to the teat canal that opens onto the tip of the teat. The teat canal is lined by a stratified squamous epithelium that is continuous with the skin. Single teat sinuses and canals pass through the teats of ruminants, while the teats of carnivores, horses, and pigs contain multiple teat sinuses and canals, each opening separately onto the surface. The skin surface of the teat of cows and pigs lacks sebaceous glands, sweat glands, and hairs.

Chestnuts and **ergots** are epidermal thickenings characteristic of the horse. The **claws** of carnivores, **hooves** of ungulates, and **horns** of ruminants are highly specialized derivatives of the skin composed of hard keratin.

CHICKEN

The **epidermis** of the chicken is generally thinner than that of mammals. It is composed of an inner **stratum germinativum** and an outer **stratum corneum.** The stratum germinativum includes a **basal layer,** an **intermediate layer** of one to several layers of polygonal cells, and a thin **transitional layer** of flat vacuolated cells just below the stratum corneum.

The **dermis** of feathered skin lacks papillae and is nonglandular. Mutlilocular, as well as unilocular, adipocytes occur in the **subcutis.**

The epidermally derived **feathers** may be classified into three main types in the adult chicken: contour, down, and filoplume. A **contour feather** has a central shaft that is divisible into a hollow **calamus** (quill) and a **rachis.** A **vane** extends laterally from each side of the rachis and is composed of **barbs** and **barbules** with interlocking **hooklets.** **Down feathers** are soft and fluffy. Their barbules lack hooklets. **Filoplumes** are small, hairlike feathers.

Feathers are situated in tubelike **follicles** oriented obliquely in the dermis or subcutis. The follicle wall of a developing feather is lined by a stratum corneum and underlying stratum germinativum surrounded by a layer of connective tissue. The **epidermal collar,** a thick ring of epidermal cells at the base of the follicle, gives rise to the feather. It surrounds the **dermal** (feather) **papilla,** which gives rise to a well-vascularized, mesenchyme-like **feather pulp** that is present during growth of the feather. A network of **feather muscles,** each composed of one to several bundles of smooth muscle, attaches the follicles to each other. No muscles are associated with the follicles of filoplumes.

Wattles and **combs** are appendages of the skin whose dermis contains an extensive, superficial network of sinus capillaries and abundant mucous connective tissue. The sinus capillaries are responsible for the striking red color of the appendages.

Digital pads are covered by a thick stratum corneum and contain a cushion of adipose tissue in their subcutis. **Scales, claws,** and **beaks** are keratinized derivatives of the skin.

The **uropygial** (preen) **gland** is a bilobed holocrine gland located in the dorsal base of the tail. It produces an oily secretion. Simple tubular glands radiate outward from the lumen of each lobe like the bristles of a bottle brush. Each tubule is divided into a **sebaceous zone** and a **glycogen zone,** named according to their histochemical staining properties. The glycogen zone is continuous with the lumen of the lobe. Each lobe is drained by a **primary duct** that passes through the **isthmus** to the **papilla** (nipple) to open onto the surface.

Figure 12.1

×12.5

Figure 12.1. Planum Nasale and Hairy Skin, Nose, Dog. Junction of the hairless planum nasale (thick skin) and the hairy portion (thin skin) of the nose. No glands are associated with the planum of carnivores. There are surface grooves in the planum of the dog.

Figure 12.2. Planum Nasale and Hairy Skin, Nose, Cat. No hairs or glands are associated with the planum of carnivores. The surface of the planum bears numerous small raised tubercles that are characteristic of the cat.

Figure 12.3. Epithelium, Planum Nasale, Cat. Portions of the small tubercles typical of the cat's planum. All layers of the epidermis are evident. Note how the papillae of the dermis interdigitate with the epidermal pegs.

Figure 12.2

×12.5

Figure 12.3

×90

Figure 12.4   ×26

Figure 12.5   ×625

KEY	
1. Dermis	6. Sebaceous gland
2. Epidermis	7. Sinus hair follicle
3. Hair follicle	8. Stratum basale
4. Intercellular bridges	9. Stratum spinosum
5. Melanocyte	10. Sweat gland

Figure 12.4. Nose, Horse. Numerous small sebaceous glands, sweat glands, fine hairs, and the follicle of a sinus hair are evident. The epidermis is heavily pigmented.

Figure 12.5. Nose, Horse. A melanocyte with numerous pigment granules is located in the deep portion of the epidermis. Surrounding cells have phagocytized melanin granules produced by melanocytes. The granules are aggregated like a cap just above the nucleus of some of the cells of the stratum spinosum.

Figure 12.6

×12.5

Figure 12.7

×250

Figure 12.8

×18

Figure 12.9

×62.5

KEY		
1. Dermal papilla		7. Nasolabial gland
2. Dermis		8. Stratum basale
3. Duct		9. Stratum corneum
4. Epidermis		10. Stratum spinosum
5. Merocrine sweat gland		11. Surface groove
6. Myoepithelial cell, nucleus		

Figure 12.6. Planum Rostrale, Pig. The very thick epidermis of the snout of the pig has low, wide elevations and an especially thick stratum corneum. Long dermal papillae project into the epidermis. Numerous merocrine sweat glands occur in the subcutis. Hairs, which are sparse on the planum of the pig, are not shown.

Figure 12.7. Planum Rostrale, Pig. Detail of the merocrine sweat glands. Secretory cells are either columnar or cuboidal and are surrounded by myoepithelial cells.

Figure 12.8. Planum Nasolabiale, Cow. The surface of the planum of the cow is hairless and marked by grooves. Long dermal papillae project into the thick epidermis. Glands are abundant in the subcutis of the planum of ruminants.

Figure 12.9. Planum Nasolabiale, Cow. The tissue was cut parallel to the surface of the planum, so that cross sections of dermal papillae appear in the stratum spinosum. Each papilla is surrounded by cells of the stratum basale and each contains several blood vessels.

Figure 12.10   ×360

Figure 12.13   ×125

Figure 12.10. Planum Nasolabiale, Cow. During tissue processing the keratinocytes of the stratum spinosum shrink away from each other, but remain attached at multiple sites where desmosomes are located. As a result of this artifact, there appear to be cytoplasmic connections between adjacent cells. Some early workers called these "intercellular bridges," because they were thought to represent cytoplasmic connections between cells. Others thought the artifacts resembled spines, hence the name stratum spinosum.

Figure 12.11. Planum Nasolabiale, Cow. The planum of the cow, sheep, and goat contains many tubuloacinar serous glands. Branches of an intralobular duct can be seen entering secretory acini.

Figure 12.12. Digital Pad, Dog. The digital pad is hairless and covered by a very thick epidermis that is roughened by small conical projections in the dog. Compare with Figure 12.14.

Figure 12.13. Digital Pad, Dog. Coiled merocrine sweat glands and pacinian corpuscles among skeletal muscle and loose connective tissue of the digital pad.

Figure 12.11   ×250

Figure 12.12   ×25

Figure 12.14

×52

Figure 12.15

×250

KEY	
1. Dermis, papillary layer	6. Stratum basale
2. Dermis, reticular layer	7. Stratum corneum
3. Digital cushion	8. Stratum granulosum
4. Duct of sweat gland	9. Stratum lucidum
5. Epidermis	10. Stratum spinosum

Figure 12.14. Digital Pad, Cat. The surface of the digital pad of the cat is smooth, lacking the conical papillae that are typical of the dog (see Fig. 12.12). Portions of the excretory ducts of sweat glands spiral through the stratified squamous epithelium.

Figure 12.15. Digital Pad, Cat. Detail of the epidermis and dermis shown in Figure 12.14. All five layers of the epidermis are evident.

Figure 12.16   ×260

KEY	
1. Dermis	4. Stratum corneum
2. Hair, x.s.	5. Stratum granulosum
3. Stratum basale	6. Stratum spinosum

Figure 12.16. Skin, Mid-Ventral Abdomen, Dog. The epidermis is thin and consists of four layers. Note that only a few layers of cells comprise the stratum spinosum. The stratum corneum is also relatively thin, and the keratinized cells have loosened and separated from the surface.

Figure 12.17

×52

Figure 12.18

×125

Figure 12.19

×125

KEY	
1. Arrector pili muscle	8. Sebaceous gland
2. Common follicular opening	9. Skeletal muscle
3. Dermis, deep	10. Stratum basale
4. Dermis, superficial	11. Stratum corneum
5. Epidermis	12. Stratum spinosum cell,
6. Hair	nucleus
7. Hair bulb	13. Subcutis

Figure 12.17. Skin, Back, Cat. Two compound follicles in the dermis. In carnivores the hairs of compound follicles merge at the level of the sebaceous glands and share a common follicular opening to the surface. Bits of hairs are evident in the follicles as shiny, yellow-brown structures. The arrector pili muscles of the skin of the back are especially well developed in cats and dogs. A space artifact separates the subcutis from the underlying skeletal muscle.

Figure 12.18. Skin, Caudal Abdomen, Cat. The epidermis is extremely thin. Cells of the stratum spinosum are sparse, and those of the stratum granulosum are visible only as occasional dark granular areas just beneath the stratum corneum. Hairs are visible within the compound follicles.

Figure 12.19. Skin, Back, Cat (Masson's). Portions of an arrector pili muscle, sebaceous gland, and a hair within a follicle.

Figure 12.20

×52

KEY	
1. Dermis	5. Hair follicle
2. Epidermis	6. Sebaceous gland
3. Hair	7. Sweat gland
4. Hair bulb	

Figure 12.20. Skin, Neck, Horse. Simple hair follicles occur in the skin of noncarnivores.

Figure 12.21

×360

Figure 12.22   ×125

Figure 12.21. Skin, Neck, Horse. Mid-region of a longitudinal section of a hair follicle. Large, clear cells of the medulla of the hair have round nuclei that become pyknotic as they progress distally from the hair bulb. The pigment-laden cortex of the hair is formed from closely packed elongated cells that have become keratinized. Scalelike, keratinized cells of the cuticle of the hair partially overlap so that their free edges point upward. They interlock with cells of the cuticle of the inner root sheath, whose free edges are directed downward.

Figure 12.22. Skin, Neck, Horse. A dermal papilla projects into the hair bulb at the base of the follicle. Cells of the cortex of the hair are nearly obscured by pigment granules provided by melanocytes of the bulb.

Figure 12.23   ×12.5

Figure 12.24   ×250

Figure 12.25   ×62.5

Figure 12.26   ×12.5

Figure 12.27   ×36

KEY	
1. Adipose tissue	9. Hair
2. Collagenous fiber	10. Hair bulb
3. Dartos muscle	11. Sebaceous gland
4. Dermis	12. Stratum basale
5. Dermis, deep layer	13. Stratum corneum
6. Dermis, superficial layer	14. Stratum granulosum
7. Elastic fiber	15. Stratum spinosum
8. Epidermis	16. Sweat gland

Figure 12.23. Skin, Dorsal Neck, Pig. Note the extremely thick dermis. Sweat glands and adipose tissue are seen in the subcutis.

Figure 12.24. Skin, Dorsal Neck, Pig. The epidermis and part of the dermis are shown in detail.

Figure 12.25. Skin, Dorsal Neck, Pig (Orcein). The dermis of the skin contains numerous branching elastic fibers. The fibers of the superficial layer are fine, while those of the deep layer are coarse.

Figure 12.26. Skin, Back, Sheep. Various portions of numerous hair follicles are embedded in the thick superficial layer of the dermis. The hair follicles of sheep tend to be arranged vertically, rather than diagonally, in the dermis. Compare with Figures 12.17 and 12.20.

Figure 12.27. Scrotum, Goat. The epidermis of the scrotum is remarkably thin. Portions of two, simple, hair follicles are located in the dermis. Bundles of smooth muscle among fibroelastic tissue in the dermis comprise the tunica dartos.

Figure 12.28 ×125

Figure 12.32 ×250

Figure 12.29 ×12.5

Figure 12.28. Scrotum, Goat. The thin epidermis and a portion of a hair follicle are shown in detail.

Figure 12.29. Pinna (Auricle), External Ear, Dog. A plate of elastic cartilage is covered by the skin of the outer (convex) and inner (concave) surfaces of the pinna. Hair follicles are more numerous in the skin of the outer surface.

Figure 12.30. Pinna, External Ear, Dog. Clusters of compound hair follicles cut in cross section vary in appearance at different levels of the dermis. The cells of the cortex and medulla of the hairs are evident in the deepest portions of the follicles. More superficially, the cells become keratinized and appear shiny pink (medulla) and yellow (cortex). Several hairs have merged to share a common follicle wall near the epidermis.

Figure 12.31. Pinna, External Ear, Dog. Detail of follicles, shown in cross section, from the deep region of the dermis, similar to those in Figure 12.30.

Figure 12.32. Skin, Back, Sheep. A wool hair, shown in cross section, lacks a medulla.

Figure 12.30 ×62.5

Figure 12.31 ×250

Figure 12.33   ×18

Figure 12.35   ×125

KEY		
1. Annular sinus	8.	Hair bulb
2. Connective tissue sheath, inner	9.	Inner root sheath
3. Connective tissue sheath, outer	10.	Merkel's cell
4. Endothelial cell, nucleus	11.	Outer root sheath
5. Epidermis	12.	Sebaceous gland
6. Erythrocytes	13.	Sinus pad
7. Hair	14.	Trabecula

Figure 12.33. Sinus Hair Follicle, l.s., Nose, Cow. In sinus hair follicles of ruminants, horses, and pigs the entire length of the blood-filled sinus is crossed by numerous trabeculae.

Figure 12.34. Sinus Hair Follicle, oblique section, Nose, Dog. The large sinus hair follicle contains a blood-filled sinus, lined by an endothelium, between the inner and outer layers of the connective tissue sheath. In carnivores only the lower region of the sinus is spanned by a network of trabeculae of connective tissue. The upper region contains an annular sinus, free of trabeculae, into which protrudes a thickening of the inner connective-tissue sheath called the sinus pad.

Figure 12.35. Sinus Hair Follicle, Nose, Dog. Detail of Figure 12.34. Portion of the sinus pad, annular sinus, and trabeculated sinus. Note the Merkel's cells, associated with tactile stimulation, in the external (outer) root sheath.

Figure 12.34   ×36

Figure 12.36   ×125

Figure 12.37   ×62.5

Figure 12.38   ×250

Figure 12.39   ×250

Figure 12.40   ×125

KEY	
1. Capillary	9. Outer root sheath
2. Duct	10. Pyknotic nucleus
3. Follicular folds	11. Sebaceous gland
4. Gland cells, surface cut	12. Secretory portion, sweat gland
5. Hair	13. Stem cell
6. Hair follicle	14. Sweat gland, l.s.
7. Inner root sheath	15. Sweat gland, x.s.
8. Myoepithelial cell, nucleus	16. Vacuolated cell

Figure 12.36. Sebaceous Gland and Hair Follicle, l.s., Lip, Sheep. The inner-root sheath forms follicular (circular) folds below the entrance of sebaceous glands into the follicle.

Figure 12.37. Nose, Dog. Longitudinal sections of two serpentine sweat glands. Their tubular structure is evident.

Figure 12.38. Sebaceous Gland and Sweat Gland, Nose, Dog. The secretory portion of a sweat gland, lined by cuboidal to columnar cells, is continuous with the bistratified, flattened cells of its duct. The cell types found in the holocrine sebaceous gland are evident: small, flat, peripheral stem cells; maturing, round cells with pale, vacuolated cytoplasm; inner degenerating cells with pyknotic nuclei.

Figure 12.39. Sweat Gland, Skin, Horse (Trichrome). Cross and oblique sections of a coiled sweat gland in the dermis are lined by cuboidal to columnar cells and surrounded by myoepithelial cells. The solid sheet of several cells represents a surface cut through the wall of the gland.

Figure 12.40. Sweat Gland and Duct, Teat, Sheep. Low columnar secretory cells with apical blebs end abruptly where the duct epithelium begins. Both the secretory cells and the initial segment of the duct are surrounded by myoepithelial cells. The cytoplasm of the myoepithelial cells appears as a pink, sometimes rippled band.

Figure 12.41 ×125

Figure 12.42 ×250

Figure 12.43 ×12.5

Figure 12.44 ×250

Figure 12.45 ×25

KEY	
1. Basement membrane	8. Hair follicle
2. Clear cell	9. Myoepithelial cell, cytoplasm
3. Dark cell	10. Myoepithelial cell, nucleus, l.s.
4. Dermis	11. Myoepithelial cell, nucleus, x.s.
5. Duct of sweat gland	12. Sebaceous gland
6. Epidermis	13. Secretory cell, nucleus
7. Hair bulb	14. Sweat gland

Figure 12.41. Sweat Gland, Teat, Sheep. The secretory cells of sweat glands vary from squamous to tall columnar. They are squamous in this preparation, but are columnar in Figure 12.40. Note that one of the secretory portions is cut tangentially, revealing the elongated shape of the myoepithelial cells.

Figure 12.42. Sweat Gland, Teat, Sheep (Silver and Eosin). The basement membrane of a sweat gland is blackened with silver. Myoepithelial cells occur between the flattened secretory cells and the basement membrane.

Figure 12.43. Carpal Gland, Pig. Lobules of merocrine sweat glands occur in the subcutaneous tissue on the medial side of the carpus of the pig.

Figure 12.44. Carpal Gland, Pig. Dark and clear cells of the secretory units of these merocrine sweat glands are surrounded by myoepithelial cells.

Figure 12.45. Infraorbital Pouch (Sinus), Sheep. Many large sebaceous glands occupy the wall of the infraorbital pouch of sheep. Some apocrine sweat glands lie deep to the sebaceous glands.

Figure 12.46

×25

Figure 12.50

×25

Figure 12.47

×12.5

KEY	
1. Corpora amylacea	8. Intralobular connective tissue
2. Epidermis	9. Intralobular duct
3. Gland	10. Lobule
4. Glandular epithelium	11. Lymphatic vessel
5. Hair follicle	12. Sebaceous gland
6. Interlobular connective	13. Secretory unit
tissue	14. Sweat gland
7. Interlobular duct	

Figure 12.46. Inguinal Pouch, Sheep. The skin of the inguinal pouch of sheep contains a few hairs, sebaceous glands, and an abundance of apocrine sweat glands.

Figure 12.47. Mammary Gland, Inactive, Cat. Lobules of glandular tissue and ducts are surrounded by fibroelastic subcutaneous tissue. The overlying skin contains a few hairs. Large lymphatic vessels lie deep to the parenchyma.

Figure 12.48. Mammary Gland, Inactive, Cow. Abundant interlobular connective tissue and components of the duct system are evident in an inactive gland. Interlobular ducts branch into the lobules as intralobular ducts.

Figure 12.49. Mammary Gland, Inactive, Cow. Lobules are composed of intralobular ducts and intralobular connective tissue, which is moderately rich in cells. Thickenings at the terminations of intralobular ducts represent remnants or precursors of glandular epithelium. When these are cut in cross section, they cannot always be distinguished from ducts.

Figure 12.50. Mammary Gland, Active, Cow. In the active gland, secretory parenchyma is well developed and connective tissue is reduced. Compare with Figure 12.48. The lumens of the secretory glands and ducts are filled with secretion *(deep pink)*.

Figure 12.48

×25

Figure 12.49

×125

Figure 12.51   ×125

Figure 12.52   ×250

Figure 12.53   ×12.5

Figure 12.54   ×62.5

Figure 12.55   ×12.5

KEY	
1. Connective tissue	7. Secretory cell, nucleus
2. Corpora amylacea	8. Secretory unit
3. Epidermis	9. Smooth muscle
4. Intralobular connective tissue	10. Sweat gland
5. Myoepithelial cell, nucleus	11. Teat sinus
6. Secretion	

Figure 12.51. Mammary Gland, Active, Cow. A portion of a lobule containing numerous tubuloacinar secretory units. Some of the alveoli contain round concretions of casein and cellular debris called corpora amylacea.

Figure 12.52. Mammary Gland, Active, Cow. Many secretory cells have basally displaced nuclei and indistinct lateral cell borders. These cells appear pale because their cytoplasmic lipids have been extracted. Sloughed cells, whose dark nuclei are visible in the lumens, are part of the secretory product. Some of the flat nuclei surrounding the alveoli belong to myoepithelial cells.

Figure 12.53. Teat, x.s., Dog. A portion of the teat shows numerous sinuses among intermingling bundles of smooth muscle and fibroelastic connective tissue. Nonruminants have multiple teat sinuses and teat canals. Some glands and hairs are associated with the skin of the teat of carnivores, horses, sheep, and goats.

Figure 12.54. Teat Sinus, x.s., Dog. Detail of a teat sinus of Figure 12.53 reveals a highly folded lining. Glandular areas, composed of small secretory units, are associated with the wall of the sinus.

Figure 12.55. Teat Sinus, x.s., Cat. This cross section through a teat reveals five teat sinuses. Some of these contain a secretion that is stained pink.

Figure 12.56 ×125

Figure 12.59 ×25

Figure 12.57 ×12.5

KEY	
1. Bistratified columnar epithelium	8. Hair follicle
2. Bistratified cuboidal epithelium	9. Lamina propria
3. Blood vessel	10. Lymphatic vessel
4. Collagenous band	11. Sebaceous gland
5. Elastic fibers	12. Smooth muscle
6. Epidermis	13. Sweat gland
7. Epithelium	14. Teat sinus

Figure 12.56. Teat Sinus, x.s., Horse (Orcein). A band of collagenous fibers lies between the epithelium and the underlying fibroelastic connective tissue.

Figure 12.57. Teat Sinus, x.s., Cow. The mucosa of the teat sinus blends with the middle layer of the teat. The latter contains well-developed, longitudinally oriented blood vessels (cut in x.s.); bundles of smooth muscle; fibroelastic tissue; and lymphatic vessels. The outer layer, the skin surface, is not shown.

Figure 12.58. Teat Sinus, x.s., Cow. The teat sinus is lined by a bistratified cuboidal to columnar epithelium.

Figure 12.59. Teat Sinus, x.s., Sheep, Male. The skin of the teat contains hairs, sebaceous glands, and sweat glands, except in the cow and pig. Compare with Figure 12.63.

Figure 12.58 ×180

Figure 12.60

×62.5

Figure 12.61

×12.5

Figure 12.62

×62.5

Figure 12.63

×25

KEY		
1. Bistratified columnar epithelium		8. Smooth muscle
2. Bistratified cuboidal epithelium		9. Stratified squamous epithelium
3. Blood vessel		10. Stratum basale
4. Dermis		11. Stratum corneum
5. Epidermis		12. Stratum spinosum
6. Epithelium		
7. Lamina propria		

Figure 12.60. Teat Sinus and Canal, Junction, x.s., Horse. Patches of the bistratified epithelium (columnar and cuboidal) of the teat sinus intermingle with the stratified squamous epithelium of the teat canal.

Figure 12.61. Teat Canal, x.s., Cow (Trichrome). The keratinized stratified squamous lining of the teat canal is encircled by a papillated layer *(green)* of connective tissue and bundles of smooth muscle *(pale yellow)*.

Figure 12.62. Teat Canal, x.s., Cow (Trichrome). Detail of the thick keratinized stratified squamous epithelium and the surrounding connective tissue and smooth muscle shown in Figure 12.61.

Figure 12.63. Skin Surface, Teat, x.s., Cow (Trichrome). The skin surface of the teat of the cow and pig is hairless.

Figure 12.64   ×26

Figure 12.65   ×12.5

Figure 12.66   ×12.5

KEY	
1. Claw fold	7. Limiting furrow
2. Dermis	8. Merocrine sweat gland
3. Digital pad	9. Middle phalanx
4. Distal phalanx	10. Sole
5. Epidermis, digital pad	11. Wall
6. Laminae	

Figure 12.64. Developing Claw, l.s., Fetus, Dog. The claw of carnivores consists of a dorsal and lateral wall (body, claw plate) and a ventral sole of hard keratin that cover the distal phalanx. The claw fold is the skin that covers the wall at the base of the claw. Endochondral bone formation has begun in the phalanges of this specimen.

Figure 12.65. Sole of Claw and Digital Pad, Dog. The limiting furrow separates the digital pad from the sole of the claw.

Figure 12.66. Apex of Claw, l.s., Dog. The dermis of the wall bears laminae (lamellae) at the apex of the claw.

Figure 12.67

×12.5

Figure 12.68

×12.5

Figure 12.69

×62.5

Figure 12.70

×125

KEY	
1. Dermal papilla	6. Stratum basale
2. Dermis	7. Stratum corneum
3. Hair follicle	8. Stratum granulosum
4. Horn tubule	9. Stratum spinosum
5. Intertubular horn	

Figure 12.67. Horn, Cow. Horns of ruminants are composed of bone of the cornual process covered by a dermis and epidermis. The epidermis with a thick stratum corneum of hard keratin (horn) and a portion of the underlying papillated dermis are shown here. (Photograph of a histologic section borrowed from the College of Veterinary Medicine, Iowa State University.)

Figure 12.68. Chestnut, Horse. Junction of the hairy skin and chestnut. Chestnuts (and ergots) of horses are keratinized thickenings of the epidermis composed of horn tubules (tubular horn) and intertubular horn. Horn tubules arise from the cells of the stratum basale that cover the apex and sides of dermal papillae. Intertubular (interpapillary) horn arises from the cells of the stratum basale that are located between the bases of the dermal papillae. Only a small portion of the very thick stratum corneum of the chestnut is shown.

Figure 12.69. Chestnut, Horse. Detail of a portion of the epidermis.

Figure 12.70. Chestnut, Horse. The section was cut parallel to the surface of the chestnut at the level of the stratum corneum. Horn tubules appear in cross section between intertubular horn.

The equine **hoof** is the keratinized portion of the epidermis that covers the distal end of the digit. The various regions of the hoof are depicted in Figures 12.71 and 12.72. The **perioplic, coronary,** and **laminar** regions comprise the wall (the portion of the hoof that is visible when the digit is on the ground). The wall turns in ventrally at an acute angle to form the **bars.** The **sole,** which forms most of the ventral surface of the hoof, is attached to the bars and the adjacent, inner border of the wall. The **frog,** a caudal, wedge-shaped mass, lies between the bars. The apex of the frog merges with the sole cranially. The **bulbs** are the convex protuberances located above and behind the frog.

The keratinized tissue comprising the hoof is in the form of **tubular, intertubular,** and **laminar horn** (see Figs. 12.75, 12.76, 12.79, and 12.80). The underlying, living layers of the epidermis include the stratum spinosum, whose cells are undergoing keratinization, and the stratum basale. The stratum basale borders on the dermis (corium), which is rich in blood vessels and nerves. The dermis may be either papillated or laminated, depending on whether the overlying epidermis contains tubular or laminated horn, respectively. The dermis blends with underlying structures such as the subcutaneous cushions and the periosteum of the third phalanx.

The **perioplic epidermis** forms a band of soft, nonpigmented tubular horn. It merges with the epidermis of the skin above and extends downward as a thin, glossy, flaky layer of keratin that forms the outer coating of the wall of the hoof, called the **stratum tectorium** (stratum externum). This layer is well developed in young animals, but tends to be worn away in older horses. The perioplic epidermis widens at the heels to form the bulbs. The **perioplic dermis**

is characterized by the presence of fine, short papillae (1 to 2 mm).

The germinal cells of the **coronary epidermis** form horn tubules (tubular horn) and intertubular horn that extend from the coronary region to the ground surface, forming the bulk of the wall of the hoof, the **stratum medium.** The horn tubules are oriented at an angle to the ground. They parallel the external surface of the hoof. The **coronary dermis** is marked by long dermal papillae (4 to 6 mm).

The **laminar epidermis** of the wall is in the form of **laminae** (lamellae) that are arranged parallel to the horn tubules of the stratum medium. They extend from the deep edge of the coronary region to the sole. Each **primary lamina** bears numerous **secondary laminae** (not present in the hooves of pigs and ruminants) that project at right angles along its length. The primary epidermal laminae are keratinized and fused with the inner portion of the stratum medium of the wall. The secondary epidermal laminae consist of a core of cells of the stratum spinosum bordered by cells of the stratum basale. The epidermal laminae form the **stratum internum** of the wall of the hoof. They interdigitate with primary and secondary dermal laminae of the **laminar dermis.** This extensive interdigitation serves to suspend the third phalanx from the hoof. At the ground surface, the junction of the epidermal laminae of the wall (unpigmented) with the sole is called the **white line.**

The tubular and intertubular horn of the bulbs, sole, and frog is softer than that of the wall of the hoof. The dermis of these regions, like that of the periople and coronary region, is papillated. The epidermis and dermis of the bars are laminated, being continuous with the laminar region of the wall.

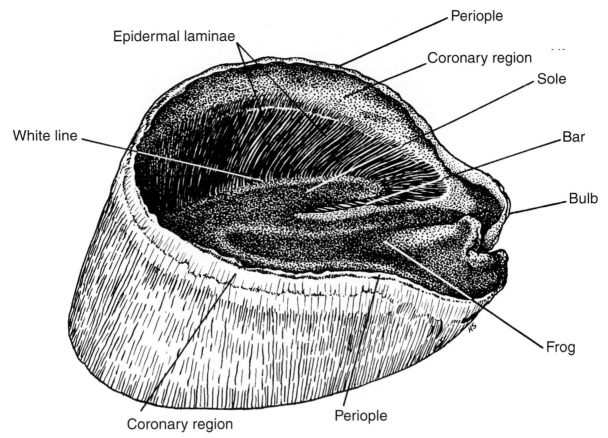

Epidermal laminae

Periople

Coronary region

Sole

Bar

Bulb

White line

Coronary region

Periople

Frog

Figure 12.71. Hoof, Horse. The various regions of the hoof are shown. The inner surface of the periople and coronary region and that of the sole, frog, and bulbs are stippled in the drawing. In the intact toe, dermal papillae extend into the funnel-shaped depressions whose openings are represented by the stipples.

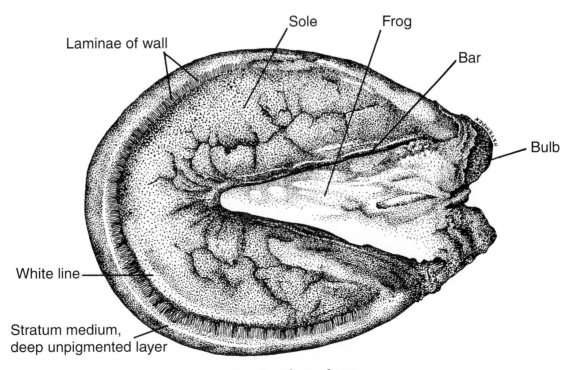

Laminae of wall

Sole

Frog

Bar

Bulb

White line

Stratum medium, deep unpigmented layer

Figure 12.72. Sole, Hoof, Horse.

Figure 12.73   ×12.5

Figure 12.74   ×25

Figure 12.75   ×125

Figure 12.76   ×12.5

Figure 12.77   ×25

KEY	
1. Bone, P_3	10. Hair follicle, developing
2. Cartilage, developing P_3	11. Horn tubule
3. Coronary dermis	12. Horn tubule, cortex
4. Coronary epidermis	13. Horn tubule, medulla
5. Dermal papilla	14. Intertubular horn
6. Dermis, sole	15. Laminar dermis
7. Dermis, wall	16. Perioplic dermis
8. Epidermis, sole	17. Perioplic epidermis
9. Epidermis, wall	

Figure 12.73. Developing Hoof, l.s., Fetus, Horse. The regions that form the three layers of the hoof wall are apparent: the perioplic, coronary, and laminar regions.

Figure 12.74. Developing Hoof, Coronary Region, l.s., Fetus, Horse. Portion of coronary epidermis and coronary dermis, later in development than in Figure 12.73, showing tubular and intertubular horn. The medulla and cortex of the horn tubules are formed from the cells of the stratum basale that cover the tip and the sides of dermal papillae, respectively. Intertubular horn is formed by cells of the stratum basale that are located between the bases of the dermal papillae. (Photograph of a histologic section borrowed from the College of Veterinary Medicine, Iowa State University.)

Figure 12.75. Developing Hoof, Coronary Region, l.s., Fetus, Horse. Detail of Figure 12.74, showing two horn tubules in longitudinal section. (Photograph of a histologic section borrowed from the College of Veterinary Medicine, Iowa State University.)

Figure 12.76. Hoof, Coronary Region, x.s., Horse. Dermal papillae and horn tubules of tubular horn. (Photograph of a histologic section borrowed from the College of Veterinary Medicine, Iowa State University.)

Figure 12.77. Developing Hoof, Wall and Sole, x.s., Fetus, Horse. The dermis of the wall is laminated, while that of the sole is papillated.

Figure 12.78

×125

Figure 12.78. Developing Hoof, Wall, x.s., Fetus, Horse. Detail of Figure 12.77. The epidermal laminae, at this time, consist mainly of a layer of basal cells (stratum basale). Primary epidermal laminae have begun to form secondary laminae. The primary and secondary dermal laminae are extensions of the laminar dermis.

Figure 12.79. Hoof, Laminar Region, x.s., Horse. Horn tubules of the stratum medium are seen in cross section. Primary and secondary epidermal laminae of the stratum internum interdigitate with the laminar dermis, which anchors the third phalanx to the wall of the hoof. Epidermal laminae, which are long ridges, appear featherlike in cross section. (Photograph of a histologic section borrowed from the College of Veterinary Medicine, Iowa State University.)

Figure 12.80. Hoof, Laminar Region, x.s., Horse. Primary epidermal laminae of the stratum internum, continuous with the stratum medium, bear secondary epidermal laminae. These interdigitate with primary and secondary dermal laminae. The secondary epidermal laminae and the dermal laminae comprise the sensitive laminae. Nuclei of the basal cells appear as small dark spots along the periphery of secondary epidermal laminae. (Photograph of a histologic section borrowed from the College of Veterinary Medicine, Iowa State University.)

Figure 12.79

×12.5

Figure 12.80

×90

Figure 12.81

×25

Figure 12.85

×250

Figure 12.82

×125

Figure 12.81. Hoof, Sole, oblique section, Horse. Dermal papillae and horn tubules of the sole are shown. (Photograph of a histologic section borrowed from the College of Veterinary Medicine, Iowa State University.)

Figure 12.82. Skin, Neck, Chicken. The epidermis of feathered skin is very thin and composed of a stratum germinativum and stratum corneum. The layers of the stratum germinativum are evident in Figure 12.92. Nuclei of the epidermal cells are often organized into stacks perpendicular to the surface. Abundant small blood vessels appear in the superficial region of the dermis.

Figure 12.83. Feather Follicle, Skin, Neck, Chicken. Oblique section through the basal region of a follicle with a developing feather. An epidermal collar surrounds the dermal papilla. The upper portion of the dermal papilla blends with the feather pulp.

Figure 12.84. Skin, Chicken. Oblique sections of developing contour feathers.

Figure 12.85. Skin, Chicken. Oblique section of a developing contour feather. Melanocytes lie among cells of the barb. Barbule cells, beginning with the outermost ones, receive pigment from the processes of the melanocytes.

Figure 12.83

×62.5

Figure 12.84

×25

Figure 12.86

×125

KEY	
1. Air space	7. Feather pulp
2. Barbules	8. Feather sheath
3. Calamus (quill)	9. Stratum corneum, follicle
4. Cells of barb stem	10. Stratum corneum, skin
5. Dermis	11. Stratum germinativum, follicle
6. Feather muscle	12. Stratum germinativum, skin

Figure 12.86. Skin, Chicken. Longitudinal section of a contour feather showing several developing barbs, later in development than in Figure 12.85. The pale, cuboidal cells at the base of each barb form the stem of the barb.

Figure 12.87. Skin, Chicken. Portion of contour feather follicle, x.s., at level of calamus (quill). Note that feather pulp has been replaced by an air space.

Figure 12.88. Skin, Chicken. Cross section of a contour feather showing numerous barbs.

Figure 12.87

×125

Figure 12.88

×90

Figure 12.89 ×90

Figure 12.92 ×250

KEY		
1. Basal layer		10. Follicle, contour feather
2. Calamus (quill)		11. Follicle, filoplume feather
3. Dermis, central layer		12. Intermediate layer
4. Dermis, superficial layer		13. Mucous connective tissue
5. Elastic tendon		14. Sinus capillary
6. Endothelial cell, nucleus		15. Stratum corneum
7. Epidermis		16. Stratum germinativum, skin
8. Erythrocyte		17. Transitional layer
9. Feather muscle		

Figure 12.89. Skin, Eyelid, Chicken. Feather follicles, x.s. The follicle wall of the tiny filoplume feather is relatively thick. A feather muscle attaches to the sheath of connective tissue of the follicle of a contour feather by an elastic tendon.

Figure 12.90. Wattle, x.s., Rooster. Numerous sinus capillaries in the superficial layer of the dermis impart a red color to the wattle (and comb) when filled with blood. Mucous connective tissue of the intermediate layer of the dermis surrounds the central layer of dense connective tissue.

Figure 12.91. Comb, Rooster. The point of a comb is similar in appearance to the wattle (see Fig. 12.90). The collagenous fibers of the central layer of the dermis arise from the periosteum of the skull and carry vessels and nerves to the extremities of the comb.

Figure 12.92. Comb, Rooster. Portion of epidermis and superficial dermis. The stratum corneum and layers of the stratum germinativum (basal, intermediate, and transitional layers) are evident. The lower ends of the cells of the basal layer bulge into the dermis, so that the epidermal-dermal boundary is uneven. Numerous anastomosing, blood-filled sinus capillaries in the superficial layer of the dermis are lined by pigment-laden endothelial cells.

Figure 12.90 ×12.5

Figure 12.91 ×12.5

Figure 12.89 ×90

Figure 12.90 ×12.5

Figure 12.91 ×12.5

Figure 12.92 ×250

Figure 12.93 ×25

KEY	
1. Adipose tissue	12. Merkel's cell
2. Blood vessel	13. Mucous connective tissue
3. Bone	14. Oral cavity
4. Dermal papilla	15. Palatine ridge
5. Dermis, central layer	16. Periosteum
6. Dermis, intermediate layer	17. Sinus capillary
7. Dermis, superficial layer	18. Sinus capillaries
8. Epidermal peg	19. Stack of nuclei
9. Epidermis	20. Stratum corneum
10. Fibroblast	21. Stratum germinativum
11. Herbst corpuscle	22. Tomial edge

Figure 12.93. Comb, Hen. The comb of a laying hen, compared with that of a rooster, contains less mucous connective tissue and more dense connective tissue in the intermediate layer, as well as fewer and smaller sinus capillaries in the superficial layer of the dermis (see Fig. 12.94).

Figure 12.94. Comb, Hen. Detail of the epidermis and a portion of the dermis in Figure 12.93. Fewer and smaller sinus capillaries are in the superficial layer of the dermis of the comb of the laying hen as compared with that of the rooster. Note the arrangement of the nuclei of epidermal cells into stacks.

Figure 12.95. Comb, Hen. Numerous Merkel's cells are located along the inner surface of the epidermis. These cells are associated with tactile nerve endings.

Figure 12.96. Upper Beak, x.s., Chicken. One side of the upper beak is shown. The bone of the premaxilla is covered by a periosteum, dermis, and epidermis with a thick layer of hard keratin. The dermis of the lateral surface of the upper beak often contains Herbst corpuscles; one corpuscle is shown here (see Fig. 9.35 for detail of this corpuscle). Dermal papillae of the lateral surface diminish medially. The lower beak slips inside the upper beak between the palatine ridge and the stratum corneum of the medial surface.

Figure 12.97. Upper Beak, x.s., Chicken. Detail of dermis and epidermis of the tomial edge of Figure 12.96. Cells of the stratum basale vary in height and width, so that intermittent groups of tall slender cells form epidermal pegs between which project dermal papillae.

Figure 12.94 ×25

Figure 12.98 ×25

KEY		
1. Adipose tissue, subcutis	5. Stratum corneum	
2. Dermis	6. Stratum germinativum	
3. Keratin, hard	7. Sulcus	
4. Keratin, soft		

Figure 12.98. Spur, Hen. The spur cap consists of an extremely thick stratum corneum of hard keratin.

Figure 12.99. Scutes, l.s., Anterior Metatarsus, Chicken. Scutes are large scales that are covered by hard keratin. Their region of overlap, shown here, forms a sulcus lined by soft keratin.

Figure 12.100. Scutes, l.s., Anterior Metatarsus, Chicken. The region of overlap of two scutes shows the transition from the hard keratin to the deeper-staining, soft keratin of the sulcus.

Figure 12.101. Reticulate Scale, x.s., Digit, Chicken. The hard keratin of the stratum corneum covers the outer surface and lines the sulci of these small scales from the lateral metatarsus.

Figure 12.102. Digital Pad, Chicken. A thick keratinized epithelium, a dermis, and a thick cushion of adipose tissue in the subcutis characterize the digital pad.

Figure 12.95 ×250

Figure 12.96 ×12.5

Figure 12.97 ×62.5

Figure 12.99 ×12.5

Figure 12.100 ×62.5

Figure 12.101 ×25

Figure 12.102 ×12.5

Figure 12.103 ×250

KEY	
1. Bone, distal phalanx	9. Sebaceous zone
2. Capsule of connective tissue	10. Stratum germinativum
3. Dermis	11. Tendon
4. Dorsal plate, claw	12. Unguinal scale, dorsal surface
5. Footpad	13. Unguinal scale, ventral surface
6. Glycogen zone	
7. Lobe, lumen	14. Ventral plate, claw
8. Multilocular fat cell, nucleus	

Figure 12.103. Multilocular Fat, Digital Pad, Chicken. Multilocular fat cells, containing numerous lipid vacuoles and a central nucleus, are common in the subcutis of the chicken.

Figure 12.104. Claw, l.s., Chicken. The dotted line indicates the approximate location of the drawing (cross section) of the claw shown in Figure 12.105.

Figure 12.105. Claw, Base, x.s., Chicken.

Figure 12.106. Claw, Base, x.s., Chicken. Compare this photomicrograph with Figures 12.104 and 12.105. The free edge of the dorsal, unguinal scale (scute type) overlaps the base of the claw, so that a cross section reveals a dorsal and ventral surface of the scale. The soft keratin of the ventral surface of the scale abuts the dorsal plate of hard keratin of the base of the claw. The dorsal plate curves ventrally over the bone of the distal phalanx.

Figure 12.107. Uropygial Gland, l.s., Chicken. A portion of one lobe of this bilobed holocrine gland shows branched tubular glands surrounded by a capsule of connective tissue. Each tubular gland is composed of a peripheral, sebaceous zone and an inner, glycogen zone. The latter communicates with the lumen of the lobe.

Figure 12.104

Figure 12.108. Uropygial Gland, l.s., Chicken. The lumen of a lobe communicates with a primary duct, which passes through the isthmus toward the papilla of the gland.

Figure 12.109. Uropygial Gland, l.s., Chicken. The two primary ducts pass through the papilla (nipple). Their openings (not shown) onto the surface are surrounded by feathers.

Figure 12.110. Sebaceous Zone, Uropygial Gland, Chicken. Portions of tubular glands are shown in cross section. The basal layer of the glandular epithelium is represented by the oval to flat nuclei of the small basal cells. A single layer of acidophilic and grainy intermediate cells lies on the basal layer. Cells of the thick, central (transitional) layer accumulate lipid, hypertrophy, and degenerate toward the luminal surface.

Figure 12.111. Glycogen Zone, Uropygial Gland, Chicken. Portions of tubular glands are shown in cross section. Intermediate cells, with an acidophilic and grainy cytoplasm, form a thick layer in the glycogen zone. The pale cells of the central layer are less numerous. Compare with Figure 12.110.

Figure 12.105

Figure 12.106   ×12.5

Figure 12.107   ×12.5

13

DIGESTIVE SYSTEM

MAMMALS

The digestive tract extends from the mouth to the anus. Generally, its wall is composed of an outer **serosa** (or an **adventitia**), **muscularis externa, submucosa,** and inner **mucosa.** The mucosa consists of an inner **epithelium,** a middle **lamina propria,** and an outer **muscularis mucosae.** A muscularis mucosac is absent from the mouth, pharynx, portions of the esophagus, and the rumen. The mouth lacks a submucosa and muscularis externa.

From the lips through the nonglandular stomach, the epithelium of the mucosa is stratified squamous. Among other places the epithelium is keratinized on the dental pad, surface of the tongue, hard palate, cheek, and the nonglandular stomach of ruminants, horses, and pigs. The epithelium of the mucosa in the glandular stomach and the intestine is simple columnar; in the anal canal it is stratified squamous.

From the mouth through the esophagus, the mucosa is moistened by the secretions (mucous or serous) of various glands, including the major salivary glands. Surface mucous cells and mucous neck cells of the stomach and goblet cells of the small and large intestines also contribute lubricating secretions.

The **tongue** has various small outgrowths, **papillae,** located primarily on its upper surface. These vary considerably in size and appearance. Some (**filiform**) have threadlike projections or bear spines. Some are cushion-shaped (**circumvallate, fungiform**), while others (**foliate**) take the form of a succession of folds. **Taste buds** occur in the epithelium of circumvallate, foliate, and fungiform papillae.

The **oropharynx** is lined by a stratified squamous epithelium and contains mucous glands, except in carnivores, where the glands are mixed. A muscularis externa of skeletal muscle is surrounded by an adventitia.

Throughout most of its length, the **esophagus** is surrounded externally by an adventitia. The muscularis externa varies in composition. In the dog it is composed of skeletal muscle throughout its length, except in the vicinity of the stomach, where skeletal muscle is replaced by smooth muscle. In ruminants the entire muscularis externa is comprised of

119

skeletal muscle. In the horse and cat a switch from skeletal to smooth muscle occurs in the caudal third of the esophagus, whereas in the pig the change occurs just cranial to the diaphragm.

The mucosa of the esophagus is lined by stratified squamous epithelium. The longitudinally arranged smooth muscle of the esophageal muscularis mucosae varies in amount from anterior to posterior. It is in the form of isolated bundles anteriorly and a continuous sheet posteriorly in the cat, horse, and ruminant. In the dog and pig it is absent anteriorly and appears as a continuous sheet posteriorly.

Mucous or **mixed glands** occur in the submucosa of the esophagus. In the cat, horse, and ruminant, glands occur only at the junction of the pharynx and esophagus. In the pig they occur anteriorly, diminish in the mid-region, and are sparse caudally. In the dog they occupy the entire length of the esophagus and extend into the stomach for a short distance.

The horse, ruminant, and pig have a nonglandular **forestomach** and a **glandular stomach**. In ruminants the forestomach is divisible into a rumen, reticulum, and omasum. The glandular stomach of ruminants is the abomasum. The cat and dog have a glandular stomach, but lack a forestomach. In all of these animals the glandular stomach consists of **cardiac, fundic,** and **pyloric gland regions.** The cardiac gland region is relatively small in all but the pig.

The epithelium of the glandular stomach invaginates into the lamina propria, forming tubular structures called **gastric pits** (foveolae). Depressions of the mucosa known as **gastric furrows** are also present.

Various **tubular glands** empty into the bottom of the gastric pits. **Mucous glands** with occasional parietal cells are the principal type found in the cardiac gland region. In the fundic gland region glands are constructed mostly of **parietal** and **chief cells,** which secrete hydrochloric acid and pepsinogen, respectively. The glands of the pyloric gland region are mainly of the mucous type with interspersed parietal cells.

In carnivores the mucosa of the fundic gland region is separated into an adoral, narrow, and thin **light zone** and an aboral, wide, and thick **dark zone.** These zones are readily visible on gross examination of the mucosa and are distinguishable histologically. The stomach of the cat has a thick layer of connective tissue between the base of the glands and the muscularis mucosae called the **stratum compactum.** This may be capped by a layer of fibroblasts, the **stratum granulosum.** The combination of these cells and the stratum compactum is called the **lamina subglandularis.** The latter may be absent in dogs. A submucosa, muscularis externa of smooth muscle, and serosa complete the wall of the stomach.

The intestines of mammals consist of a **small intestine** (duodenum, jejunum, and ileum) and a **large intestine** (cecum, colon, rectum, and anal canal). In both the small and large intestine, the epithelium is simple columnar with a **striated border. Goblet cells** occur among the columnar cells. The former increase in number from anterior to posterior with the greatest number occurring in the large intestine.

Villi are confined to the small intestine in mammals. They are short and thick in ruminants but long and slender in carnivores. At the bases of the villi are invaginations of the epithelium, the **crypts of Lieberkühn** (intestinal glands). Replacement of the mucosal epithelium occurs by cell division primarily within the crypts. A muscularis mucosae, consisting of two layers of smooth muscle, separates the crypts from the underlying submucosa. The latter is formed from loose connective tissue in the horse, ruminant, and pig. In contrast, it is composed of moderately dense connective tissue in carnivores. A **lamina subglandularis** may be present in the intestine of carnivores. The remainder of the wall of the intestine is comprised of a muscularis externa of smooth muscle and a serosa.

Compound, tubuloacinar **Brünner's glands** (duodenal glands, submucosal glands) are mucous glands occurring within the submucosa and often within the lamina propria of the duodenum. In carnivores, sheep, and goats they are limited to the initial or mid-region of the duodenum; in horses, pigs, and cows they extend into the jejunum. Brünner's glands also project into the pyloric stomach for a short distance. Aggregations of lymphatic nodules, **Peyer's patches,** are present in the lamina propria and submucosa of the small intestine, especially the ileum.

The mucosa of the **large intestine** presents a flat surface. Villi are absent. Crypts are longer than in the small intestine. Flat bands, **taenia coli,** consisting of longitudinally arranged smooth muscle and elastic fibers, occur in the colon of horses and pigs. Similar structures, **taenia ceci,** occur in the cecum. The **rectum** terminates at the **anal canal,** which is lined by a stratified squamous epithelium. The epithelium is nonkeratinized in the anterior portion of the canal and keratinized in the posterior portion, which is continuous with the hairy skin. Tubuloacinar **anal glands** occur in the submucosa and muscularis of the anal canal in carnivores and pigs. **Circumanal glands** occur in the subcutis around the anus of the dog. The upper portion of these glands is sebaceous, whereas the lower portion is nonsebaceous. The cells of the latter resemble hepatocytes. Accordingly, the nonsebaceous region is often called a **hepatoid gland.**

Paired **anal sacs** occur lateral to and below the anus of carnivores. Each is lined by a keratinized, stratified squamous epithelium and is located between the inner smooth muscle of the internal anal sphincter and the outer skeletal muscle of the external anal sphincter. The excretory duct of each gland opens into the keratinized portion of the anal canal. **Glands of the anal sac** are apocrine tubular in the dog. In the cat both apocrine tubular glands and sebaceous glands surround the anal sac.

The **liver** is a large, lobed gland. Each lobe is covered by a mesothelium, beneath which is a thin connective-tissue layer, the **capsule of Glisson.** Each lobe is divided into numerous **classic lobules.** These consist of **sinusoids** and of plates of parenchyma cells, **hepatocytes,** radially organized about a central vein. Lobules are indistinctly separated from one another in all animals except the pig, in which an abundance of connective tissue between lobules clearly identifies their boundaries. **Portal tracts** (areas) occur at the interstices of three or more lobules. Each tract contains one or more branches of a portal vein, hepatic artery, bile ductule, and lymphatic vessel. These various components are supported by a framework of connective tissue.

Bile, secreted by hepatocytes, enters tiny bile canaliculi from which it flows into the canals of Hering, located close to each portal tract. The canals unite with the bile ductule of a portal tract. Bile ductules lead into bile ducts. The epithelium of bile ductules is simple cuboidal, whereas that of the bile ducts is simple columnar. **Goblet cells** occur in the largest bile ducts.

The **gallbladder** is a storage depot for bile. Its mucosa is thrown into numerous folds when the bladder is contracted. When it is distended, they mostly disappear. The simple columnar epithelial lining has a striated border. Goblet cells have been reported in the epithelium of the cow. We have also observed them in the goat. Mucous, serous, or mixed glands are often seen in the wall of the gallbladder of ruminants. The smooth muscle of the muscularis is arranged circularly (mostly oblique, according to some) for the most part. The gallbladder is absent in the horse.

The **pancreas** consists of numerous tubuloacinar secretory units, which form the exocrine component of the organ. Clusters of epithelial cells, the endocrine **islets of Langerhans,** are scattered among the secretory units. Tubuloacinar units drain into long, narrow **intercalated ducts,** which are lined by elongated cells that present a cuboidal appearance when sectioned transversely. Intercalated ducts communicate directly with **interlobular ducts.** Striated (secretory) ducts are not present. Unlike salivary glands, myoepithelial cells are lacking around the secretory units. **Pacinian corpuscles** are commonly found within the connective tissue of the pancreas of dogs and cats.

CHICKEN

In the chicken the **salivary glands** are all of the mucous variety. They are located in the roof and floor of the oral cavity, tongue, and pharynx. **Taste buds** are present but sparse. They are associated with the ducts of salivary glands at the base of the tongue and the pharynx.

The **esophagus** has the usual seven layers. It is lined by a thick, nonkeratinized, stratified squamous epithelium. The muscularis externa is composed of smooth muscle along the entire length of the esophagus. Mucous glands occur in the lamina propria, but are lacking throughout most of the **crop,** which is a caudal diverticulum located approximately two-thirds of the way down the esophagus. The crop has a structure identical to the rest of the esophagus, but it lacks mucous glands.

The **stomach** of the chicken consists of a glandular **proventriculus** and a muscular **ventriculus** (gizzard). The mucosa of the proventriculus is thrown into folds (plicae).

Depressions between the folds are called sulci. The epithelium is simple columnar except at the base of the sulci, where it is cuboidal. The wall of the proventriculus consists of large, compound, tubular glands. The secretory cells, which are cuboidal to low columnar, produce both pepsinogen and hydrochloric acid, thus combining the function of mammalian chief and parietal cells. Each gland opens to the lumen of the stomach through a conical papilla.

The ventriculus is a highly muscular grinding organ. It is lined by an epithelium that invaginates into the lamina propria, forming elongated pits, each of which bears terminal tubular gastric glands. Cells of the latter secrete a thick, horny material. Although keratin-like, this substance, usually called keratinoid, is not chemically equivalent to keratin. It forms the tough inner lining, about 1 mm thick, of the ventriculus.

The **intestine** of the chicken is similar in structure throughout its length. It consists of a **duodenum, jejunum, ileum,** and **large intestine.** A pair of blind, elongated **ceca** join the intestine at the junction of the ileum and large intestine. The terminal end of the large intestine joins the coprodeum of the **cloaca.** Villi are present throughout the small and large intestines. They are longest in the duodenum, but gradually shorten and thicken caudally. In the coprodeum they are stumpy and rounded. Villi are present in the ceca also, becoming flattened toward the blind end. **Crypts of Lieberkühn** are short and open between the villi, as in mammals. Although the wall of the intestine of the chicken is similar to that of the mammal, the absence of duodenal glands and an extremely thin submucosa in the chicken are notable differences.

As in mammals, the **liver** is covered by a mesothelium beneath which is a layer of connective tissue, **Glisson's capsule.** Lobes of the liver are subdivided into numerous lobules indistinctly separated from one another. The radiating plates of hepatocytes in each lobule are two cells wide in the chicken. In contrast, those of mammals are one cell wide.

The **gallbladder** of the chicken is similar to that of the mammal. The mucosa is lined by a simple columnar epithelium and is strongly folded into villuslike projections when contracted.

The **pancreas** of the chicken resembles that of the mammal. The exocrine portion is tubuloacinar. Lobulation is indistinct because of the lack of interlobular connective tissue. Islets of Langerhans are abundant. Two types of islets, alpha and beta, can be easily recognized. Columnar alpha cells characterize the alpha islet. Polygonal beta cells are the principal cells of the beta islets. Alpha islets produce glucagon, whereas beta islets form insulin.

Figure 13.1   ×25

Figure 13.5   ×12.5

Figure 13.2   ×25

KEY	
1. Alveolar bone	11. Mucous acinus
2. Connective tissue, papilla of	12. Outer enamel epithelium
3. Dental lamina	13. Sebaceous gland
4. Dental papilla	14. Serous acinus
5. Dental sac	15. Serous demilune
6. Duct	16. Skeletal muscle
7. Hair follicle	17. Stellate reticulum
8. Inner enamel epithelium	18. Stratified squamous
9. Intralobular duct	epithelium, keratinized
10. Labial gland	19. Stratum granulosum

Figure 13.1. Lip, Sheep. The section was taken through the junction of the hairy and nonhairy portions of the lip. The stratum granulosum is present in the epidermis of the hairy portion of the lip, but disappears at the junction with the nonhairy portion of the lip. Portions of hair follicles are present.

Figure 13.2. Lip, Sheep. Oral surface of the lip with mixed labial glands among the skeletal muscle.

Figure 13.3. Lip, Sheep. Mixed labial glands within the skeletal musculature.

Figure 13.4. Cheek, Sheep. The mucous membrane of the cheek of ruminants is characterized by numerous, conical papillae. The apex and lateral surfaces of the papillae are highly keratinized.

Figure 13.5. Developing Permanent Tooth, Dog. The ectodermally derived enamel organ has differentiated into the outer and inner enamel epithelium and the stellate reticulum. The dental papilla, derived from mesenchyme, is in contact with the inner enamel epithelium.

Figure 13.3   ×125

Figure 13.4   ×12.5

Figure 13.6   ×12.5

Figure 13.6. Developing Permanent Tooth, Dog. Dentin and enamel formation has begun (see Fig. 13.7).

Figure 13.7. Dentinoenamel Junction, Developing Permanent Tooth, Dog. Odontoblasts cover the surface of the mesenchymal dental papilla. These cells produce predentin (uncalcified dentin). The pale layer of predentin abuts the recently calcified dentin. The enamel organ consists of tall, columnar ameloblasts that produce enamel; a stratum intermedium; and the stellate reticulum.

Figure 13.8. Root of Tooth, x.s., and Periodontal Ligament, Dog. The periodontal ligament consists of bundles of collagenous fibers, blood and lymphatic vessels, nerves, and cells (mostly fibroblasts). The fiber bundles extend between, and anchor to, the cementum of the tooth and the alveolar bone. The ends of the fibers that are embedded in either cementum or bone are called Sharpey's fibers. They are indistinct in this micrograph.

Figure 13.9. Upper Deciduous Tooth, Decalcified, and Gingiva, l.s., Dog. The enamel space identifies the location of enamel before it was lost during decalcification. The attachment (junctional) epithelium of the gingiva is nonkeratinized stratified squamous and lacks papillae of connective tissue. It abuts the enamel region and is continuous with the papillated, keratinized stratified squamous epithelium of the free gingiva.

Figure 13.7   ×125

Figure 13.8   ×62.5

Figure 13.9   ×25

Figure 13.10   ×12.5

Figure 13.11   ×62.5

Figure 13.12   ×25

Figure 13.13   ×25

Figure 13.14   ×12.5

KEY		
1. Adipose tissue	8.	Palatine bone
2. Connective tissue, papilla of	9.	Stratified squamous epithelium, keratinized
3. Horn tubule-like structure		
4. Lamina propria	10.	Stratum basale
5. Loose connective tissue	11.	Stratum corneum
6. Mixed gland	12.	Stratum spinosum
7. Mucous gland	13.	Submucosa

Figure 13.10. Dental Pad, Cow. The dental pad of ruminants is distinguished by its thick stratum corneum and well-developed papillae of connective tissue.

Figure 13.11. Epithelium, Dental Pad, Sheep. The section shows a thick stratum corneum and underlying stratum spinosum. A horn, a tubulelike structure, extends through the stratum corneum.

Figure 13.12. Hard Palate, Caudal, Dog (Masson's). All domestic mammals, except the pig, have glands (mucous or mixed) in the submucosa of the caudal portion of the hard palate. The cranial portion lacks glands in all of the domestic mammals.

Figure 13.13. Hard Palate, Pig. Large irregular patches of pale, loose connective tissue are scattered throughout the submucosa.

Figure 13.14. Soft Palate, Cow. Mucous glands and adipose tissue occupy portions of the lamina propria and submucosa. The epithelium is stratified squamous and keratinized.

Figure 13.15   ×52

Figure 13.16   ×25

Figure 13.17   ×25

Figure 13.18   ×250

KEY	
1. Connective tissue, papilla of	7. Skeletal muscle
2. Connective tissue, papilla of (caudal)	8. Small papilla
3. Connective tissue, papilla of (rostral)	9. Spine
4. Filiform papilla, projection of	10. Stratum spinosum
5. Fungiform papilla, core	11. Supporting cell, nucleus
6. Sensory cell, nucleus	12. Taste pore

Figure 13.15. Filiform Papilla, Tongue, Cat. The filiform papilla of carnivores contains several, small, rostral papillae of connective tissue and a large, caudal papilla of connective tissue. A large, keratinized spine is associated with the caudal papilla.

Figure 13.16. Filiform Papillae, Tongue, Horse. In horses and pigs delicate, threadlike, keratinized projections extend from the upper surfaces of the filiform papillae. The papillae of connective tissue are long, but are not subdivided.

Figure 13.17. Fungiform and Filiform Papillae, Tongue, Goat. This section is from the tip of the tongue. The fungiform papilla is moundlike in section with a broad, core of connective tissue containing numerous nerves. Portions of keratinized filiform papillae appear on either side. In ruminants the connective tissue of filiform papillae is subdivided into several small papillae.

Figure 13.18. Taste Bud, Fungiform Papilla, Tongue, Horse. The taste bud is embedded within the keratinized stratified squamous epithelium of a fungiform papilla. Supportive and sensory cells are visible within the bud. The nucleus and cytoplasm of the sensory cells are slightly darker than those of the supporting cells.

Figure 13.19

×52

KEY	
1. Connective tissue, core of	4. Lingual salivary gland
2. Connective tissue, papilla of	5. Stratified squamous epithelium
3. Duct	6. Taste buds

Figure 13.19. Circumvallate Papilla, Tongue, Goat. This large papilla lies within a depression of the lingual epithelium. Taste buds occur within the epithelium of the papilla facing the cavity of the depression, but are usually absent from the upper surface of the papilla.

Figure 13.20 ×25

Figure 13.21 ×25

Figure 13.22 ×36

Figure 13.23 ×25

KEY	
1. Adipose tissue	9. Muscle, longitudinal
2. Core of connective tissue	10. Muscle, transverse
3. Filiform papilla	11. Muscle, vertical
4. Interlobular connective tissue	12. Serous gland
5. Interlobular duct	13. Skeletal muscle
6. Intralobular duct	14. Stratified squamous
7. Lobule	epithelium, keratinized
8. Mucous gland	15. Space artifact

Figure 13.20. Conical Papilla, Tongue, Goat. This highly keratinized papilla is located on the upper surface of the tongue.

Figure 13.21. Lingual Salivary Glands, Horse. Both mucous and serous glands occur between the skeletal muscle bundles of the tongue.

Figure 13.22. Musculature, Tongue, l.s., Cat. The vertical, horizontal, and transverse arrangement of the lingual skeletal musculature can be seen below the mucosal papillae.

Figure 13.23. Parotid Gland, Horse. Portions of several lobules are shown. Lobules are often delineated by space artifacts. See Fig. 13.24 for detail of a lobule.

Figure 13.24 ×250

Figure 13.28 ×250

Figure 13.24. Parotid Gland, Horse. Serous acini, intercalated ducts, and striated (secretory) ducts are present. The latter show clearly defined basal striations.

Figure 13.25. Parotid Gland, Dog. Serous acini and intralobular ducts are shown.

Figure 13.26. Parotid Gland, Cow. The secretory units are lined by pale, acidophilic cells with large nuclei. The cells vary in height, giving the luminal surface a scalloped appearance. This feature is unique to the cow.

Figure 13.27. Submandibular Gland, Dog. Mucous acini (some with serous demilunes) and serous acini characterize the parenchyma.

Figure 13.28. Submandibular Gland, Sheep. Intercalated ducts branching from a striated duct.

Figure 13.25 ×125

Figure 13.26 ×250

Figure 13.27 ×125

Figure 13.29

×250

Figure 13.29. Submandibular Gland, Sheep (Mallory's). The junction between a mucous acinus and an intercalated duct is illustrated.

Figure 13.30. Sublingual Gland, Dog. In the cat, dog, and horse the sublingual gland contains mucous secretory units, serous acini, and serous demilunes. Long tubular mucous units are a characteristic feature of the gland in the dog.

Figure 13.30

×130

Figure 13.31 ×125

Figure 13.33 ×12.5

KEY	
1. Adipose tissue	8. Interlobular connective tissue
2. Blood vessel	9. Mixed glands
3. Coat of connective tissue	10. Mucous acinus
4. Duct	11. Serous demilune
5. Epithelium	12. Skeletal muscle
6. Goblet cells	13. Stratified squamous epithelium
7. Intercalated duct	14. Striated duct

Figure 13.31. Sublingual Gland, Pig. In the pig and ruminant, mucous tubuloacinar secretory units predominate. Serous demilunes are sparse.

Figure 13.32. Interlobular Duct, Sublingual Gland, Pig. This large interlobular duct is lined by a columnar epithelium. In places the latter is bistratified. Goblet cells occur in the epithelium.

Figure 13.33. Oropharynx, Dog. The section shows mixed glands among the skeletal muscle and within the submucosa. Mixed glands are shown in detail in Figure 11.10.

Figure 13.32 ×90

Figure 13.34

×62.5

Figure 13.34. Oropharynx, Dog (Orcein). A thick band of connective tissue, containing numerous elastic fibers, parallels the mucosa.

Figure 13.35. Esophagus, Mid-Region, x.s., Dog. The glands of the dog's esophagus are predominantly mucous. They are located in the submucosa throughout the length of the esophagus of the dog. The muscularis externa is skeletal muscle, except very near the stomach (see Fig. 13.36).

Figure 13.35

×52

Figure 13.36

×62.5

Figure 13.36. Esophagus, Near Stomach, l.s., Dog. The muscularis externa of the dog's esophagus is composed of skeletal muscle, except in the region caudal to the diaphragm, where the musculature is mixed.

Figure 13.37. Esophagus, Cranial, l.s., Cat. A few mixed glands are present in the submucosa. In the cat, horse, and ruminant, esophageal glands occur only near the junction of the esophagus and pharynx. The stratified squamous lining of the esophagus of carnivores is typically nonkeratinized. In the cat and horse the muscularis externa is skeletal muscle throughout much of the esophagus. The transition from skeletal to smooth occurs in the caudal one-fifth to one-third of the esophagus in these animals.

Figure 13.38. Esophagus, Cranial, x.s., Horse. The papillated stratified squamous epithelium shows a distinct keratinized layer. The epithelium is also keratinized in pigs and ruminants. A sparse muscularis mucosae is present in the cranial esophagus in the horse, cat, and ruminant. The muscularis externa consists of skeletal muscle in this region.

Figure 13.39. Esophagus, Cranial, l.s., Pig. The stratified squamous epithelium is also keratinized in horses and ruminants. Note the abundance of mucous glands in the submucosa. In the cranial portion of the esophagus, a muscularis mucosae is absent in the pig and dog. The muscularis externa consists of skeletal muscle in this region.

Figure 13.37

×25

Figure 13.38

×12.5

Figure 13.39

×12.5

Figure 13.40

×12.5

KEY	
1. Adipose tissue	9. Muscularis externa, outer
2. Adventitia	oblique
3. Connective tissue, papilla of	10. Muscularis mucosae
4. Esophagus, lumen	11. Serosa
5. Lamina propria	12. Skeletal muscle
6. Mucous gland	13. Smooth muscle
7. Muscularis externa, inner	14. Stratified squamous
circular	epithelium, keratinized
8. Muscularis externa, outer	15. Submucosa
longitudinal	

Figure 13.40. Esophagus, Mid-Region, l.s., Pig. Note the decrease in glandular tissue and the presence of a muscularis mucosae. Compare with Figure 13.39. The muscularis externa consists of skeletal muscle in this region.

Figure 13.41. Esophagus, Caudal, x.s., Pig. The region of the pig's esophagus just cranial to the diaphragm shows the presence of smooth and skeletal muscle in the muscularis externa, a lack of glands, and a thick muscularis mucosae.

Figure 13.42. Esophagus, Caudal, x.s., Pig. Detail of Figure 13.41 shows the smooth and skeletal musculature of the muscularis externa.

Figure 13.43. Esophagus, Mid-Region, x.s., Sheep. The muscularis mucosae is less developed than in the pig (see Fig. 13.40).

Figure 13.41

×12.5

Figure 13.42

×62.5

Figure 13.43

×62.5

Figure 13.44

Figure 13.45   ×25

Figure 13.46   ×12.5

Figure 13.47   ×125

Figure 13.48

KEY	
1. Arteriole	7. Muscularis externa
2. Capillary	8. Stomach contents
3. Connective tissue, band of	9. Stratified squamous epithelium,
4. Keratinized cells	keratinized
5. Lamina propria	10. Submucosa
6. Lymphatic vessel	

Figure 13.44. Rumen, Sheep. The mucosa of the rumen is differentiated into paddle-shaped papillae.

Figure 13.45. Rumen, Cow. A part of the wall from the lumen to the beginning of the muscularis externa (smooth muscle). A complete short papilla and a portion of a long papilla are included. Note the submucosa entering the long papilla. A muscularis mucosae is not present in this part of the forestomach.

Figure 13.46. Rumen, Sheep. Section shows two cuts through adjacent long papillae. These papillae are flat, paddlelike, structures (see Fig. 13.44). The bottom one in the photograph was cut parallel to the flat surface, and the top one was cut perpendicular to the flat surface. A dense, more darkly stained band of connective tissue mimics a muscularis mucosae.

Figure 13.47. Rumen, Sheep. Section illustrates the vacuolated, keratinized cells of the stratified squamous epithelium of a papilla. Numerous capillaries abut the epithelium.

Figure 13.48. Reticulum, Sheep. The mucosa of the reticulum is extended into intersecting folds that subdivide the surface into distinct compartments suggesting a honeycomb. Conical papillae project from the crests of the folds and from the mucosa of the compartments.

Figure 13.49   ×25

Figure 13.53   ×25

Figure 13.50   ×12.5

KEY	
1. Conical papilla	5. Muscularis mucosae
2. Connective tissue, band of	6. Stratified squamous epithelium, keratinized
3. Lamina propria	
4. Muscularis externa	7. Submucosa

Figure 13.49. Reticulum, Cow. Short folds and the base of a long fold are visible. A muscularis mucosae occurs in the upper segment of the long fold. This is a characteristic feature of the reticulum. Sides and crests of long folds have conical papillae with keratinized tips.

Figure 13.50. Reticulum, Sheep. Section shows a long fold cut in a plane parallel to its flat surface. The apparent gaps are the result of undulations in the fold. Conical papillae are evident along the crest of the fold.

Figure 13.51. Reticulum, Goat (Masson's). The section is through the region of intersection of three long folds. The muscularis mucosae passes from one fold to another at the intersection. Two conical papillae, with keratinized tips, project from the sides of two of the folds.

Figure 13.52. Omasum, Sheep. Laminae (folds) of different sizes extend from the wall of the omasum somewhat like the pages of a book. The mucosal surfaces of the laminae are studded with numerous conical papillae.

Figure 13.53. Omasum, Sheep. Small folds such as the one shown contain a lamina propria and muscularis mucosae, but lack an extension of smooth muscle from the muscularis externa.

Figure 13.51   ×25

Figure 13.52

Figure 13.54 ×62.5

Figure 13.55 ×25

Figure 13.56 ×125

Figure 13.57 ×12.5

Figure 13.58 ×62.5

KEY	
1. Cardiac gland region	9. Muscularis mucosae
2. Cardiac glands	10. Papilla
3. Columnar epithelium, stomach	11. Smooth muscle of muscularis externa
4. Elastic fiber	12. Stratified squamous epithelium, esophagus
5. Fundic gland region	
6. Lamina propria	13. Stratified squamous epithelium, keratinized
7. Lymphatic vessel	
8. Mixed glands	14. Vein

Figure 13.54. Omasum, Sheep. The base of a long fold is shown. In addition to the muscularis mucosae, smooth muscle from the muscularis externa projects into the center of the fold.

Figure 13.55. Omasum, Sheep. Portions of two long folds are shown. Numerous small papillae cover the surface of the folds.

Figure 13.56. Omasum, Goat (Orcein). The lamina propria of a portion of a small papilla contains an extensive network of elastic fibers.

Figure 13.57. Junction, Esophagus and Cardiac Gland Region of Stomach, Dog. Numerous glands, predominantly mucous with a few serous demilunes, occupy the submucosa of the esophagus and extend into the cardiac gland region of the stomach of dogs.

Figure 13.58. Junction, Esophagus and Cardiac Gland Region of Stomach, Dog. Detail of Figure 13.57. The stratified squamous epithelium of the esophagus ends abruptly where the columnar epithelium of the stomach begins.

Figure 13.59   ×12.5

Figure 13.63   ×250

Figure 13.60   ×25

Figure 13.61   ×25

Figure 13.62   ×62.5

KEY	
1. Cardiac glands	9. Lamina propria
2. Cardiac sphincter	10. Lymphatic nodule
3. Chief cell	11. Muscularis mucosae
4. Connective tissue, papilla of	12. Parietal cell
5. Esophageal glands	13. Simple columnar epithelium
6. Fundic gland region	14. Stratified squamous
7. Fundic glands	epithelium, keratinized
8. Gastric pit	15. Submucosa

Figure 13.59. Junction of Esophagus and Stomach, Dog. Section passes through the cardiac sphincter.

Figure 13.60. Margo Plicatus, Horse. At the margo plicatus the keratinized stratified squamous epithelium of the forestomach ends, and the simple columnar epithelium of the cardiac gland region of the stomach begins.

Figure 13.61. Cardiac Gland Region, Stomach, Pig. Numerous lymphatic nodules characterize the mucosa of the cardiac gland region of the pig's stomach.

Figure 13.62. Light Zone, Fundic Gland Region, Stomach, Dog. The light zone of the carnivore's fundic stomach has a thinner mucosa than the more aboral dark zone. The gastric pits of the light zone are comparatively deep, extending, in some cases, to a depth equivalent to half the thickness of the mucosa. Compare with Figure 13.65. Note that smooth muscle *(arrows)* of the muscularis mucosae of the stomach extends into the lamina propria.

Figure 13.63. Light Zone, Fundic Gland Region, Stomach, Dog. Chief and parietal cells form the walls of the fundic glands. The glands are shown in cross section.

Figure 13.64   ×12.5

Figure 13.65   ×62.5

Figure 13.66   ×62.5

Figure 13.67   ×62.5

Figure 13.68   ×250

KEY	
1. Chief cells	9. Muscularis mucosae
2. Fundic gland, lumen	10. Parietal cells
3. Fundic glands	11. Serosa
4. Gastric pit	12. Smooth muscle
5. Lamina propria	13. Stratum compactum
6. Mucosa	14. Stratum granulosum
7. Mucous neck cells	15. Submucosa
8. Muscularis externa	16. Surface mucous cells

Figure 13.64. Dark Zone, Fundic Gland Region, Stomach, Dog. A portion of the stomach wall, including the base of a fold, is shown.

Figure 13.65. Dark Zone, Fundic Gland Region, Stomach, Dog. The mucosa of the dark zone of the fundic stomach of carnivores is thicker than that of the light zone. The gastric pits are comparatively shallow, extending no farther into the mucosa than one-third of its thickness. Compare with Figure 13.62.

Figure 13.66. Dark Zone, Fundic Gland Region, Stomach, Dog (PAS). The surface mucous cells lining the lumen, cells of the gastric pits and the mucous neck cells of the glands both contain complex carbohydrates and are PAS positive (magenta stain).

Figure 13.67. Lamina Subglandularis, Fundic Gland Region, Stomach, Cat (old). A thick layer of connective tissue, the stratum compactum, and an overlying layer of fibroblasts, the stratum granulosum, together form the lamina subglandularis, a structure seen consistently in cats and occasionally in dogs. Presumably, the lamina subglandularis protects the stomach from punctures by sharp objects.

Figure 13.68. Fundic Gland Region, Stomach, Cat. The fundic glands have been cut longitudinally. They are formed largely from parietal and chief cells.

Figure 13.69 ×12.5

Figure 13.70 ×62.5

Figure 13.71 ×125

Figure 13.72 ×25

Figure 13.73 ×62.5

KEY	
1. Adipose tissue	8. Mucosa
2. Cardiac glands	9. Mucous precursor
3. Chief cells	10. Muscularis externa
4. Epithelial cells, surface cut	11. Muscularis mucosae
5. Fundic glands	12. Parietal cells
6. Gastric pit	13. Simple columnar epithelium
7. Lamina propria	14. Submucosa

Figure 13.69. Fundic Gland Region, Stomach, Horse. Note the thick mucosa and submucosa.

Figure 13.70. Junction of the Cardiac and Fundic Gland Regions, Stomach, Horse. The mucous glands of the cardiac gland region are distinct from the parietal and chief cells of the fundic gland region of the stomach.

Figure 13.71. Fundic Gland Region, Stomach, Horse. A unique feature of the surface epithelium of the glandular stomach is the presence of a mucous precursor that fills the apical region of the cells.

Figure 13.72. Fundic Gland Region, Abomasum, Sheep. The submucosa shows extensive infiltration by adipose tissue.

Figure 13.73. Fundic Gland Region, Abomasum, Goat. Parietal and chief cells of the glands are evident. Note the deep gastric pits.

Figure 13.74   ×250

Figure 13.78   ×62.5

Figure 13.75   ×62.5

Figure 13.74. Fundic Gland Region, Abomasum, Cow. Parietal and chief cells of the fundic glands.

Figure 13.75. Mucosa, Pyloric Gland Region, Stomach, Dog (PAS). The content of the surface mucous cells and that of the secretory units of the pyloric glands are PAS positive *(magenta color)*.

Figure 13.76. Surface Mucous Cells, Pyloric Gland Region, Stomach, Dog. Columnar cells lining the gastric pits and bordering the gastric lumen show typical cup-shaped concentrations of mucous precursor in their apical ends. The epithelium contains many migrating lymphocytes.

Figure 13.77. Pyloric Gland Region, Stomach, Cat. Note the deep gastric pits. Some extend halfway through the thickness of the mucosa.

Figure 13.78. Mucosa, Pyloric Gland Region, Stomach, Cat. Note the presence of deep gastric pits. Some extend to about half the depth of the mucosa.

Figure 13.76   ×125

Figure 13.77   ×25

Figure 13.79   ×250

Figure 13.80   ×25

Figure 13.81

Figure 13.82   ×36

KEY	
← Junction, pyloric gland region and duodenum	7. Muscularis externa
	8. Muscularis mucosae
1. Arteriole	9. Pyloric gland
2. Brünner's gland	10. Stratum compactum
3. Crypt of Lieberkühn	11. Stratum granulosum
4. Gastric furrow	12. Submucosa
5. Gastric pit	13. Villus of duodenum
6. Lamina propria	

Figure 13.79. Pyloric Gland Region, Stomach, Cat. Basal ends of pyloric glands and the stratum granulosum and stratum compactum of the lamina subglandularis are present in this section.

Figure 13.80. Pyloric Gland Region, Abomasum, Goat. Gastric furrows and gastric pits can be seen.

Figure 13.81. Junction, Pyloric Gland Region and Duodenum, l.s., Dog. Brünner's glands are located primarily in the submucosa of the duodenum. They also extend a short distance into the pyloric gland region of the stomach. They occasionally break through the muscularis mucosae and extend into the lamina propria.

Figure 13.82. Junction, Pyloric Gland Region and Duodenum, l.s., Dog. Gastric pits and mucous glands of the pyloric gland region of the stomach can be seen. Brünner's glands (mucous) occur below the interrupted muscularis mucosae. See Figure 13.83 for detail of the epithelium.

Figure 13.83   ×260

KEY	
1. Central lacteal	5. Lymphocytes
2. Goblet cell	6. Striated border
3. Intestinal absorptive cells	7. Surface mucous cells, stomach
4. Lamina propria	

Figure 13.83. Junction, Pyloric Gland Region and Duodenum, Dog. Note the change in the epithelium when it passes from the stomach to the duodenum. Typical columnar surface mucous cells of the pyloric gland region of the stomach contrast with the columnar absorptive cells and goblet cells of the duodenum.

Figure 13.84 ×125

Figure 13.85 ×25

Figure 13.86 ×62.5

Figure 13.87 ×125

KEY			
1. Artifact		7. Muscularis mucosae	
2. Brünner's gland		8. Secretory unit	
3. Crypt of Lieberkühn		9. Serosa	
4. Duct		10. Submucosa	
5. Goblet cell		11. Villus	
6. Muscularis externa			

Figure 13.84. Brünner's Gland, Duodenum, l.s., Dog. Detail of mucous secretory units. The latter, in the dog, are lined by tall columnar cells and have large lumens. Compare with Figure 13.90.

Figure 13.85. Duodenum, x.s., Cat. A segment of the wall of the duodenum is shown. The intestinal villi of carnivores tend to be longer than those of noncarnivores. Note the shrinkage artifact at the apical ends of the villi.

Figure 13.86. Duodenum, Proximal, x.s., Cat (Masson's). Ducts of Brünner's glands penetrate the muscularis mucosae. Brünner's glands are marked off into distinct lobules in the cat.

Figure 13.87. Duodenum, x.s., Cat (Masson's). The submucosa in the cat and dog is a moderately dense irregular connective tissue. In other domestic mammals it is a loose connective tissue.

Figure 13.88   ×250

Figure 13.92   ×125

Figure 13.89   ×250

Figure 13.90   ×125

Figure 13.91   ×25

KEY	
1. Adipose cell	8. Mucous gland
2. Adipose tissue	9. Muscularis externa
3. Crypt of Lieberkühn	10. Paneth cell
4. Globular leukocyte	11. Secretory unit
5. Lamina propria	12. Serous gland
6. Lymphocyte	13. Striated border
7. Mucosa	14. Submucosa

Figure 13.88. Epithelium of Villus, Duodenum, Cat. Lymphocytes can be seen migrating through the simple columnar epithelium. Note the presence of several globular leukocytes.

Figure 13.89. Duodenum, Horse. Paneth cells are visible in the basal portions of the crypts of Lieberkühn in the small intestine of the horse.

Figure 13.90. Duodenum, Horse. In the horse, Brünner's glands have both mucous and serous components. Note that the lumens of the secretory units are small. Compare with Figure 13.84.

Figure 13.91. Duodenum, Pig. Brünner's glands fill the entire submucosa.

Figure 13.92. Duodenum, Pig. In the pig the lumens of the secretory units of Brünner's glands are very small.

Figure 13.93   ×12.5

Figure 13.97   ×125

Figure 13.94   ×125

Figure 13.93. Duodenum, l.s., Cow. Brünner's glands are present throughout much of the submucosa of an intestinal fold (plica).

Figure 13.94. Duodenum, Cow. Detail of Brünner's gland. In the cow some gland cells have an acidophilic cytoplasm. The lumens of secretory units are large.

Figure 13.95. Duodenum, x.s., Sheep. The muscularis externa of the intestine is arranged into an inner circular and an outer longitudinal layer of smooth muscle. Compare the appearance of the muscle layers seen in this cross section with that of the longitudinal section of the intestine in Figure 13.96.

Figure 13.96. Duodenum, l.s., Sheep. This section is through the muscularis externa. Compare the appearance of the muscle layers in this preparation with that in Figure 13.95.

Figure 13.97. Duodenum, Goat. Portions of the mucosa and submucosa. The lumens of the secretory units of Brünner's glands are large in the goat.

Figure 13.95   ×125

Figure 13.96   ×125

Figure 13.98   ×62.5

Figure 13.99   ×125

Figure 13.100   ×25

Figure 13.101   ×125

Figure 13.102   ×250

KEY	
1. Auerbach's plexus	11. Muscularis externa, inner circular
2. Central lacteal, x.s.	12. Muscularis externa, outer longitu-
3. Columnar epithelium	dinal
4. Crypt of Lieberkühn	13. Muscularis mucosae
5. Eosinophil	14. Nuclei of epithelium cut obliquely
6. Globular leukocyte	15. Stratum compactum
7. Goblet cell	16. Submucosa
8. Intestinal lumen	17. Villus
9. Lamina propria	
10. Meissner's plexus	

Figure 13.98. Jejunum, x.s., Dog. A Meissner's plexus is present in the periphery of the submucosa. An Auerbach's plexus is wedged between the inner circular and outer longitudinal layers of the muscularis externa.

Figure 13.99. Jejunum, Dog. A well-developed stratum compactum is present between the lamina propria and muscularis mucosae of the small intestine in some cats and dogs.

Figure 13.100. Jejunum, x.s., Cat. Slender villi and well-defined crypts of Lieberkühn are evident.

Figure 13.101. Jejunum, Cat. Transverse sections of villi. Central lacteals are evident in two of them. Migrating lymphocytes are visible within the epithelium.

Figure 13.102. Jejunum, Cat. Globular leukocytes are present among the columnar cells lining a crypt of Lieberkühn. Numerous eosinophils are scattered through the lamina propria.

Figure 13.103   ×12.5

Figure 13.104   ×25

Figure 13.105   ×250

Figure 13.106   ×12.5

Figure 13.107   ×62.5

KEY	
1. Crypt of Lieberkühn	8. Muscularis externa, inner circular
2. Eosinophil	9. Muscularis externa, outer
3. Goblet cell	longitudinal
4. Lamina propria	10. Muscularis mucosae
5. Lymphatic nodule	11. Serosa
6. Mitotic figure	12. Submucosa
7. Mucosa	13. Villus

Figure 13.103. Jejunum, l.s., Horse. All layers of the wall are included in this section. The villi are shorter than those of carnivores.

Figure 13.104. Ileum, x.s., Cat. A portion of the wall from the lumen to the serosa is shown. The epithelium of the villi contain numerous goblet cells.

Figure 13.105. Ileum, Dog. Mitotic figures can be seen in the crypts.

Figure 13.106. Cecum, Tip, Dog. Large lymphatic nodules are present in the submucosa.

Figure 13.107. Cecum, Dog. Numerous goblet cells in the lining of the crypts of Lieberkühn are characteristic of the organ. The epithelial cells bordering the lumen in this preparation have undergone some autolysis and look tattered.

Figure 13.108   ×250

Figure 13.112   ×12.5

Figure 13.109   ×12.5

Figure 13.108. Cecum, Dog. Several crypts of Lieberkühn appear in cross section. A striated border is present on the columnar cells. Goblet cells are numerous.

Figure 13.109. Cecal Band, x.s., Horse. A cecal band consists of an admixture of smooth muscle (thickened outer longitudinal layer of the muscularis externa) and elastic fibers. Elastic fibers are predominant in the bands of both the cecum and the ventral large colon of the horse. Compare with Figure 13.112.

Figure 13.110. Cecum, Horse. Veins with bands of smooth muscle in their walls are common in the submucosa throughout the digestive tract of the horse. Similar vessels are shown at low magnification in Figure 13.109.

Figure 13.111. Cecum, Cow. In the large intestine of ruminants the crypts of Lieberkühn are usually tortuous. Adipose tissue is abundant in the submucosa.

Figure 13.112. Taenia Coli, Small Colon, x.s., Horse. The taenia coli are thickenings of the outer longitudinal layer of the muscularis externa. In contrast to the bands of the cecum and ventral large colon, where elastic fibers are predominant, smooth muscle predominates in the bands of the small colon and dorsal large colon. Compare with Figure 13.109.

Figure 13.110   ×62.5

Figure 13.111   ×25

Figure 13.113 ×12.5

Figure 13.117

Figure 13.114 ×25

KEY	
1. Adipose tissue	12. Mucosa
2. Anal canal	13. Muscularis externa, inner
3. Anal glands	circular
4. Anal sac	14. Muscularis externa, outer
5. Circumanal glands	longitudinal
6. Crypt of Lieberkühn	15. Muscularis mucosae
7. Epidermis	16. Rectum
8. External anal sphincter	17. Striated border
9. Glands of anal sac	18. Submucosa
10. Goblet cell	19. Taenia coli
11. Lamina propria	

Figure 13.113. Taenia Coli, Colon, x.s., Pig. The muscular taenia coli is formed from the outer longitudinal layer of the muscularis externa. The submucosa is infiltrated with fat.

Figure 13.114. Spiral Colon, x.s., Goat. The mucosa contains both tortuous and straight crypts of Lieberkühn. The muscularis externa shows an abrupt thickening of its inner circular layer and outer longitudinal layer.

Figure 13.115. Spiral Colon, x.s., Goat. The columnar epithelial cells have a distinct striated border.

Figure 13.116. Rectum, x.s., Cat. The epithelium of the rectum presents a flat, uniform surface.

Figure 13.117. Rectoanal Junction, l.s., Dog. Note that the anal glands mark the junction *(arrow)* of the rectum and anal canal.

Figure 13.115 ×250

Figure 13.116 ×62.5

Figure 13.118 ×12.5

Figure 13.122 ×62.5

Figure 13.119 ×125

KEY	
1. Anal gland	8. Mucosa
2. Apocrine tubular gland	9. Muscularis externa, inner
3. Circumanal gland	circular
4. Crypt of Lieberkühn	10. Sebaceous gland
5. Debris in anal sac	11. Stratified squamous
6. External anal sphincter	epithelium
7. Keratinized epithelium of	
anal sac	

Figure 13.118. Rectoanal Junction, l.s., Dog. Note the change between the stratified squamous epithelium of the anal canal and the crypts of Lieberkühn of the rectal mucosa. Note also that anal glands are located in the submucosa and are scattered among the smooth muscle of the internal anal sphincter (inner circular layer of the muscularis externa). See Figure 13.117 for orientation.

Figure 13.119. Anal Glands, Dog. Section is through the secretory units of an anal gland.

Figure 13.120. Glands of the Anal Sac, Dog. A small portion of the wall of an anal sac and the secretory units of some of the glands of the anal sac are shown. See Figure 13.117 for location.

Figure 13.121. Anal Sac, Cat. About one-half of the wall of an anal sac is shown.

Figure 13.122. Glands of the Anal Sac, Cat. Portions of these glands are shown adjacent to the skeletal muscle of the external anal sphincter. The presence of sebaceous glands in this location is a characteristic of the cat.

Figure 13.120 ×62.5

Figure 13.121 ×12.5

Figure 13.123   ×125

Figure 13.124   ×25

Figure 13.125   ×125

Figure 13.126   ×25

Figure 13.127   ×62.5

KEY	
1. Circumanal gland, nonsebaceous	8. Sebaceous gland
2. Circumanal gland, sebaceous	9. Simple columnar
3. Crypt of Lieberkühn	epithelium
4. Goblet cell	10. Skeletal muscle
5. Hair follicle	11. Stratified squamous
6. Keratinized epidermis	epithelium
7. Lamina propria	12. Stratum granulosum

Figure 13.123. Anal Canal, l.s., Dog. Junction of the keratinized and nonkeratinized regions of the anal canal. The stratum granulosum of the keratinized region stops abruptly at the junction.

Figure 13.124. Circumanal Glands, Dog. Numerous nonsebaceous portions of circumanal glands are present subcutaneously among the skeletal muscle of the anal sphincter. These nonsebaceous portions are often called hepatoid glands because their cells resemble hepatocytes.

Figure 13.125. Circumanal Gland, Dog. Detail of a part of one of the glands. The lower, nonsebaceous portion of these glands is more acidophilic than the upper, sebaceous portion.

Figure 13.126. Rectoanal Junction, l.s., Horse. The stratified squamous epithelium of the anal canal contrasts with the rectal mucosa.

Figure 13.127. Rectoanal Junction, Horse. The abrupt change between the stratified squamous epithelium of the anal canal and the simple columnar epithelium of the rectal mucosa is apparent.

Figure 13.128   ×25

Figure 13.129   ×125

Figure 13.130   ×125

Figure 13.131   ×62.5

Figure 13.132   ×900

KEY		
1. Bile canaliculus, l.s.	8.	Lobule (portion of)
2. Bile canaliculus, x.s.	9.	Lymphatic vessel
3. Bile ductule	10.	Nucleus of hepatocyte
4. Central vein, l.s.	11.	Portal vein, branch
5. Central vein, x.s.	12.	Serosa
6. Hepatic artery, branch	13.	Sinusoid
7. Hepatocyte		

Figure 13.128. Liver, Cat. Transverse and longitudinal sections through the central veins of two classic lobules.

Figure 13.129. Liver, Cat. Transverse section through a classic lobule. Sinusoids empty into the central vein. Hepatocytes radiate as hepatic plates from the central vein.

Figure 13.130. Liver, Cat. The portal tract in this section includes a branch of the hepatic portal vein and hepatic artery, bile ductule, and lymphatic vessel.

Figure 13.131. Liver, Horse. A portal tract is at the intersection of three classic lobules. Branches of the portal vein can be seen extending between the lobules.

Figure 13.132. Liver, Cat (Masson's). Sections through various bile canaliculi are evident in this section.

Figure 13.133 ×250

Figure 13.134 ×250

Figure 13.135 ×25

Figure 13.136 ×250

Figure 13.137 ×250

KEY			
1.	Bile duct	7.	Hepatocyte
2.	Binucleate hepatocyte	8.	Kupffer cell
3.	Capsule of Glisson	9.	Mesothelium
4.	Central vein	10.	Portal tract
5.	Connective tissue, partition of	11.	Portal vein, branch
6.	Goblet cell	12.	Sinusoid

Figure 13.133. Liver, Horse. A sinusoid joins with a branch of the portal vein.

Figure 13.134. Liver, Horse. Section is through mesothelial cells and connective tissue of the capsule of Glisson surrounding the liver. Together, the mesothelial cells and the capsule of Glisson comprise the serosa.

Figure 13.135. Liver, Pig. Classic lobules are clearly separated from one another by partitions of connective tissue in the pig.

Figure 13.136. Liver, Pig. Particulate-laden Kupffer cells within sinusoids of a classic lobule are evident in this section. Binucleate hepatocytes can also be seen.

Figure 13.137. Liver, Goat. A large bile duct with columnar epithelium and goblet cells.

Figure 13.138 ×36

Figure 13.139 ×250

Figure 13.140 ×25

Figure 13.141 ×250

Figure 13.142 ×125

KEY		
1. Adventitia	8.	Liver
2. Dark cell	9.	Mucosa
3. Epithelium	10.	Mucous acinus
4. Gallbladder, lumen	11.	Muscularis
5. Goblet cell	12.	Serous acinus
6. Lamina propria	13.	Striated border
7. Light cell		

Figure 13.138. Gallbladder, Dog. A portion of the wall showing the highly folded mucosa.

Figure 13.139. Gallbladder, Dog. Epithelial lining with light and dark columnar cells.

Figure 13.140. Gallbladder and Liver, Pig (Masson's). Section shows a portion of the liver and gallbladder.

Figure 13.141. Gallbladder, Goat. Portion of a mucosal fold showing goblet cells in the epithelium.

Figure 13.142. Gallbladder, Goat. Mixed glands occur within the wall of the gallbladder of ruminants.

Figure 13.143   ×125

Figure 13.147   ×250

Figure 13.144   ×25

Figure 13.143. Cystic Duct, Pig. The epithelium is composed of light cells, dark cells, and goblet cells.

Figure 13.144. Pancreas, Horse. The organ is divided into lobules by septa of connective tissue. Most of the pancreas is formed from exocrine acinar cells. Islets of Langerhans are scattered through the exocrine region of the gland.

Figure 13.145. Pancreas, Horse. Portions of two lobules showing acinar cells, interlobular ducts, and intercalated (intralobular) ducts.

Figure 13.146. Pancreas, Horse. An islet of Langerhans with some surrounding exocrine acini. In the horse the darker, A cells are located in the center of the islet, while the lighter B cells are positioned in the periphery. Compare with Figure 13.150. Note the numerous capillaries among cords of islet cells.

Figure 13.147. Pancreas, Dog. Detail of acini and intercalated ducts. Note acidophilic apical regions and basophilic basal regions of the acinar cells.

Figure 13.145   ×125

Figure 13.146   ×250

Figure 13.148   ×125

Figure 13.152   ×62.5

Figure 13.149   ×250

KEY	
1. A cell	7. Hyaline cartilage
2. Acinus	8. Intercalated duct
3. B cells	9. Islet of Langerhans
4. Centroacinar cell	10. Salivary gland
5. Duct	11. Stratified squamous epithelium
6. Goblet cell	12. Taste bud

Figure 13.148. Pancreas, Pig. An interlobular duct with goblet cells interspersed among the epithelial cells of the duct.

Figure 13.149. Pancreas, Cow (Masson's). An intercalated duct enters an acinus.

Figure 13.150. Pancreas, Sheep (Masson's). In ruminants darkly stained A cells are located at the periphery of the islets of Langerhans, while light-staining B cells are centrally located. Compare with Figure 13.146.

Figure 13.151. Tongue, Tip, l.s., Chicken. The upper surface of the tongue is covered by a thick stratified squamous epithelium, which is keratinized near the tip. The stratified squamous epithelium of the lower surface is thinner and also keratinized rostrally. The tongue is supported by hyaline cartilage rostrally. The ducts of salivary glands (mucous) open at the lower surface.

Figure 13.152. Taste Bud, Tongue, Base, Chicken. A taste bud (characteristically large and scarce in the chicken) can be seen closely associated with the duct of a salivary gland. For detail of the taste bud see Figure 13.153.

Figure 13.150   ×250

Figure 13.151   ×12.5

Figure 13.153 ×250

Figure 13.157 ×62.5

Figure 13.154 ×25

Figure 13.155 ×25

Figure 13.156 ×12.5

KEY	
1. Gland	10. Proventriculus, lumen
2. Intercellular space	11. Secondary duct
3. Lamina propria	12. Serosa
4. Mucous gland	13. Stratified squamous epithelium
5. Muscularis externa	14. Submucosa
6. Muscularis mucosae	15. Sulcus
7. Plica	16. Taste bud cell
8. Pore	17. Tertiary duct
9. Primary duct	

Figure 13.153. Taste Bud, Chicken. Detail of the taste bud seen in Figure 13.152. Its cells stain lightly with eosin. Numerous spaces occur between cells. A taste bud pore is visible.

Figure 13.154. Esophagus, x.s., Chicken. The esophagus is lined by a thick nonkeratinized stratified squamous epithelium. Mucous glands occur in the lamina propria. The submucosa is sparse.

Figure 13.155. Crop, Chicken. The crop is a diverticulum of the esophagus. Unlike the latter, it lacks mucous glands, except close to its junction with the esophagus.

Figure 13.156. Proventriculus (Glandular Stomach), x.s., Chicken. The submucosa contains lobules of compound tubular glands that are arranged around a central, secondary duct. A primary duct, which drains several lobules, opens through a raised mucosal papilla.

Figure 13.157. Proventriculus, x.s., Chicken. A magnified view of Figure 13.156 shows that the mucosa of the papilla is arranged into folds (plicae) covered by columnar cells, and depressions (sulci) lined by shorter cells. A primary duct, lined by columnar cells, joins the lumen of the proventriculus.

Figure 13.158 ×250

Figure 13.161 ×250

Figure 13.159 ×36

Figure 13.158. Proventriculus, x.s., Chicken. A tertiary duct branching from the secondary duct leads into a glandular unit. The glandular epithelial cells vary from simple cuboidal to low columnar and contain a grainy secretory material. These cells secrete both pepsinogen and HCl.

Figure 13.159. Ventriculus (Gizzard), Chicken. The pink, thick layer of keratinoid that lines the ventriculus is produced by branched tubular gastric glands in the lamina propria. The submucosa and a portion of the smooth muscle layers of a thick muscularis externa are shown.

Figure 13.160. Ventriculus, Chicken. Keratinoid lines the mucosal surface and fills the lumen of the gastric pits and glands. The cells of the surface epithelium are low to tall columnar. The cells decrease in height as they extend into the gastric pits. Flattened cells (chief cells) line the upper and mid-regions of the tubular gastric glands seen in this micrograph. Branching of some of the glands is evident.

Figure 13.161. Ventriculus, Chicken. The flattened chief cells lining the mid-portion of the gastric glands become cuboidal to low columnar in the fundus of the gland. A few, large basal cells with pale nuclei and pale cytoplasm occur in the fundus of the glands.

Figure 13.160 ×125

Figure 13.162   ×12.5

Figure 13.165   ×62.5

Figure 13.163   ×25

Figure 13.166   ×25

KEY	
1. Crypt of Lieberkühn	5. Serosa
2. Lymphatic tissue	6. Submucosa
3. Muscularis externa	7. Villus
4. Muscularis mucosae	

Figure 13.162. Duodenum, x.s., Chicken. Lymphatic tissue (diffuse and nodular) in the duodenum close to the stomach.

Figure 13.163. Duodenum, x.s., Chicken (Mallory's). The serosa is thick. The submucosa is characteristically sparse.

Figure 13.164. Ileum, x.s., Chicken. Villi are long and slender with numerous goblet cells. The submucosa is thin.

Figure 13.165. Cecum, Tip, l.s., Chicken. In the tip of the cecum, villi are short and broad. Compare Figure 11.51 of the cecal tonsil.

Figure 13.166. Large Intestine, x.s., Chicken. Villi are present in the chicken's large intestine.

Figure 13.164   ×36

Figure 13.167

Figure 13.167. Cloaca, l.s., Chicken. The cloaca is subdivided into three regions: the coprodeum, urodeum, and proctodeum. The large intestine is continuous with the coprodeum. The ureters and genital ducts terminate in the urodeum. The terminal proctodeum opens to the exterior through the cloacal lips.

Figure 13.168. Coprodeum, Cloaca, Chicken. The mucosa of the coprodeum is thrown into short, flat villi. Shallow crypts of Lieberkühn open at their bases. Simple columnar epithelium covers their surface.

Figure 13.169. Cloaca, l.s., Chicken. Branched tubular glands (modified crypts) form a part of the lymphoglandular ridge of Jolly located in the dorsal proctodeum. The epithelium of the ridge consists of tall columnar cells. A portion of the stratified squamous epithelium of the inner surface of the ventral cloacal lip can be seen.

Figure 13.170. Cloaca, l.s., Chicken. A large Herbst corpuscle lies beneath the stratified squamous epithelium of the cloacal lip. These corpuscles occur, typically, close to the latter's point of juncture with the simple columnar epithelium of the proctodeum.

Figure 13.168   ×62.5

Figure 13.169   ×62.5

Figure 13.170   ×62.5

Figure 13.171   ×36

Figure 13.172   ×250

Figure 13.173   ×250

Figure 13.174   ×125

Figure 13.175   ×250

KEY		
1. A cells		6. Erythrocytes
2. Acinus		7. Hepatocyte
3. B cells		8. Lobule, margin of
4. Capillary		9. Reticular fibers
5. Central vein		10. Sinusoid

Figure 13.171. Liver, Chicken. Central veins of several lobules are evident. One lobule is indicated by a dashed line.

Figure 13.172. Liver, Chicken. Sinusoids can be seen entering a central vein. Radiating plates of hepatocytes are two cells thick in the chicken.

Figure 13.173. Liver, Chicken (Silver). The wall of a central vein and surrounding cords of hepatocytes (whose cellular features are indistinct in this preparation) are supported by a network of reticular fibers that have been blackened with silver.

Figure 13.174. Pancreas, Chicken. Numerous portions of tubuloacinar serous glands surround an alpha islet of Langerhans. Alpha islets consist primarily of columnar A cells and a few D cells and are larger than beta islets. Erythrocytes in capillaries can be seen between cords of islet cells.

Figure 13.175. Pancreas, Chicken. Beta islets contain polygonal B cells and some D cells and are smaller than alpha islets.

14

URINARY SYSTEM

MAMMALS

The urinary system of mammals is comprised of the paired kidneys, renal pelvises, ureters, urinary bladder, and urethra.

The **kidneys** are highly vascularized, compound tubular glands that function to maintain the composition of body fluids at a constant level and to remove excretory wastes. Each kidney is surrounded by a **capsule** of connective tissue, which may contain a distinct layer of smooth muscle in its deepest portion, as in the cow, sheep, and goat. Both the cortex and medullary regions of the kidney are formed principally of numerous, closely packed, uriniferous tubules. The spaces between tubules are mainly occupied by an extensive capillary network. The cortex and medulla are arranged into one or more pyramidal configurations called renal pyramids; the apex of each pyramid is called a renal papilla. In the **cortex,** groups of radially arranged tubules form the **pars radiata** (cortical ray or medullary rays), consisting of collecting tubules and straight portions of nephrons. The **pars convoluta** (cortical labyrinth) are located between the rays and consist of renal corpuscles and numerous proximal and distal convoluted tubules. The **proximal convoluted tubules** are longer than the **distal convoluted tubules** and comprise the major portion of the cortex. Proximal convoluted tubules are distinguished by the **brush borders** of their epithelial cells and the somewhat scalloped appearance of the apical surface of their cells when the latter are seen in profile. Distal convoluted tubules have a smooth internal surface, and their cells lack a brush border.

Filtrate processed by the nephrons is passed to **collecting tubules,** which open either directly or indirectly via calyces into the **renal pelvis** through **papillary ducts** at the tip of a **renal papilla.** The epithelial cells of the collecting tubules are pale and vary from cuboidal near the distal tubules to columnar close to the papilla. Cell boundaries are normally clearly defined compared with the cells of the proximal and distal convoluted tubules. As they progress toward the renal papilla, the collecting tubules become wider. The terminal portion of these tubules is lined by a columnar or pseudostratified epithelium and is called the **papillary duct.**

Each **renal corpuscle** consists of a **Bowman's capsule** and **glomerulus**. The outer layer of Bowman's capsule is the **capsular** (parietal) **epithelium**, a simple squamous layer. The inner layer is the **glomerular** (visceral) **epithelium**. It is formed from highly branched podocytes that surround the capillary loops of the glomerulus. In most histologic preparations made for light microscopy, it is not possible to distinguish podocytes from the adjacent endothelial cells of the capillary loops. The cavity between the capsular and glomerular layers is the **urinary space**. The latter is continuous with the lumen of a proximal convoluted tubule at the urinary pole of each corpuscle. At the opposite, vascular pole an afferent and efferent arteriole unite with the capillaries of the glomerulus. A portion of the distal convoluted tubule is positioned between the afferent and efferent arterioles. The **macula densa** of the **juxtaglomerular apparatus** forms a part of the wall of the distal convoluted tubule in this region. Each macula is composed of closely grouped epithelial cells and is easily identified by the tightly packed nuclei of these cells. **Juxtaglomerular cells** are modified, cells of smooth muscle in the walls of afferent arterioles close to the glomerulus. They have an epithelioid appearance when seen in cross section.

The **medulla** of each kidney is formed from collecting tubules, thick and thin segments of the **loops of Henle,** and numerous **vasa rectae. Thick descending portions** of Henle's loop are continuations of the proximal convoluted tubules and are located close to the corticomedullary junction. They are straight tubules whose cells are lined by a brush border. Each thick descending tubule joins abruptly with a **thin segment** whose wall is formed from flattened cells with round, bulging nuclei. The straight, **thick ascending portion** of each loop resembles the distal convoluted tubule with which it is continuous.

The walls of the renal pelvis, ureter, urinary bladder, and urethra include a mucosa, muscularis of smooth muscle, and adventitia. A submucosa may be present. The lining of the mucosa is almost exclusively transitional epithelium. The hilus region, between the capsule of the kidney and the outer wall of the renal pelvis, contains loose connective tissue and adipose tissue.

The mucosa of the **ureter** presents a folded appearance. Its transitional epithelium is separated from the muscularis by a lamina propria. Tubuloalveolar mucous glands occur in the lamina propria of the first several centimeters of the ureter of the horse. A submucosa is lacking in the ureter. The muscularis consists of inner longitudinal, middle circular, and outer longitudinal layers. An adventitia of loose connective tissue surrounds the muscularis.

The transitional epithelial cells of the **urinary bladder** become flattened when the bladder is distended with urine. A lamina propria and submucosa are present. Usually, there is a thin muscularis mucosae between these layers. The muscularis, external to the submucosa, is composed of an outer and inner longitudinal and a thick middle circular layer. The inner and outer longitudinal layers may be incomplete in some areas. Much of the bladder (body and apex) is covered by a serosa. An adventitia of loose connective tissue is present at the neck of the bladder.

CHICKEN

The urinary system of the chicken consists of large, elongated, paired kidneys. Ureters drain each kidney and open into the urodeum of the cloaca. There is no renal pelvis or urinary bladder in the bird. Each kidney is partitioned into a cranial, middle, and caudal subdivision. Each subdivision is comprised of lobules. A lobule consists of a large cortical and a smaller medullary component. All of the lobules that drain into a single branch of the ureter constitute a lobe.

There are two types of nephrons. The **cortical** (reptilian) **type** is more numerous and lacks a loop of Henle. It is located entirely within the cortex. The other is the less numerous **medullary** (mammalian) **type**. It has a loop of Henle (also called a medullary loop), which extends into the medulla. Cortical nephrons are arranged radially around **central** (intralobular) **veins** of the cortex. Their renal corpuscles lie approximately midway between the intralobular vein and a peripheral interlobular vein. The cortical nephron has a smaller renal corpuscle than the medullary nephron. The large renal corpuscles of medullary nephrons lie close to the medulla. Other than size, there is no structural difference between small and large renal corpuscles. Each glomerulus contains a compact mass of **mesangial cells** (small cells with large nuclei) at its center. The mass appears basophilic because of the relatively high concentration of nuclear material. A layer of podocytes, with large round or oval nuclei, covers the surface of the glomerular capillaries, forming the **glomerular epithelium** of Bowman's capsule. The **capsular** (parietal) **layer** of Bowman's capsule consists of a simple squamous epithelium. **Juxtaglomerular cells** and a **macula densa** are associated with the renal corpuscle at its vascular pole.

Generally, cortical tissue located between renal corpuscles and interlobular veins consists mainly of proximal convoluted tubules, and that located between renal corpuscles and intralobular veins is comprised of distal convoluted tubules. Cells of proximal convoluted tubules are low columnar and have a well-developed brush border. Distal convoluted tubules are shorter than proximal convoluted tubules. Their cuboidal cells lack a brush border, but the apex may form a projecting bleb of clear cytoplasm that fills much of the lumen. In cortical nephrons a short intermediate tubule (which is without a brush border, and which is about half the diameter of a distal convoluted tubule) connects proximal convoluted tubules to distal convoluted tubules. In medullary nephrons long or short Henle's (medullary) loops connect proximal convoluted tubules to distal convoluted tubules. The thin segment of a medullary loop forms only a part of the descending limb. Hence, thin segments are less numerous than either thick descending or thick ascending portions of the loop. The diameter of a thin segment is about one-half that of a thick segment. The cells of the thin segment are cuboidal and do not stain as intensely as the cuboidal cells of the thick segments. Apical cytoplasmic blebs of the cells of the thick segments project into the lumen. **Collecting tubules** occur in the more peripheral parts of the cortex. They are lined by pale cells with cuboidal to low columnar shape and are intermediate in size between proximal convoluted and distal convoluted tubules. Collecting tubules join distal convoluted tubules to **perilobular collecting ducts**. The latter unite with those of other lobules to form **medullary tracts**, each of which is surrounded by a thin, capsule of connective tissue. Tracts group together to form a **medullary cone**. Each cone terminates in a single branch of the ureter. Cones and tracts contain thin and thick segments of medullary loops, in addition to collecting ducts. The lining epithelium of the smallest collecting ducts is simple cuboidal. It gradually becomes simple columnar and finally changes to pseudostratified columnar in the proximity of the ureteral branch.

The **ureter** of the chicken is a muscular duct about 2 mm in diameter. Its wall consists of a mucosa, muscularis, and adventitia. It is generally lined by a pseudostratified columnar epithelium. The majority of cells are tall with a lesser number of cuboidal cells lying close to the basement membrane. The apices of the columnar cells contain numerous vacuoles filled with mucus. Beneath the epithelium is a thick layer of loose connective tissue containing varying amounts of diffuse lymphatic tissue and, sometimes, a lymphatic nodule. The muscularis consists of an inner longitudinal and outer circular layer of smooth muscle. A third outer longitudinal layer is present near the cloaca. The adventitia consists of a layer of loose connective tissue.

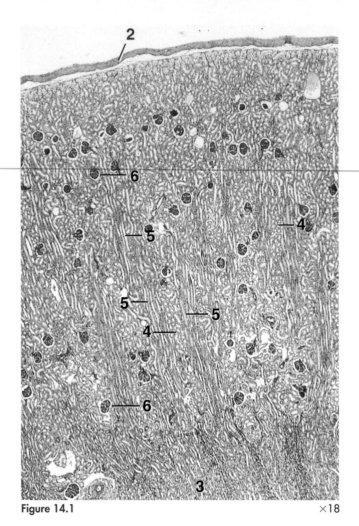

Figure 14.1   ×18

Figure 14.2   ×36

KEY	
1. Adipose tissue	4. Pars convoluta
2. Capsule	5. Pars radiata
3. Medulla	6. Renal corpuscle

Figure 14.1. Cortex and Portion of Medulla, Kidney, Dog. Renal corpuscles are limited to the cortex.

Figure 14.2. Cortex, Kidney, Dog (Masson's). Pars radiata alternate with the pars convoluta.

Figure 14.3

×125

Figure 14.4

×250

Figure 14.5

×250

Figure 14.6

×250

KEY	
1. Capsular epithelium	7. Glomerular epithelium
2. Capsule	8. Macula densa
3. Collecting tubule	9. Proximal convoluted tubule
4. Connective tissue	10. Smooth muscle
5. Distal convoluted tubule	11. Subcapsular vein
6. Fat vacuole	12. Urinary space

Figure 14.3. Capsule and Superficial Cortex, Kidney, Cat. The capsule consists entirely of connective tissue in the cat.

Figure 14.4. Capsule, Kidney, Sheep. The inner portion of the capsule of ruminants contains a distinct layer of smooth muscle. Smooth muscle is also present in the capsule of the dog, horse, and pig.

Figure 14.5. Renal Corpuscle, Kidney, Puppy. In young animals the podocytes of the glomerular epithelium have round to oval nuclei.

Figure 14.6. Renal Corpuscle, Kidney, Cat. Cells of the proximal convoluted tubules of the cat contain numerous fat vacuoles. A macula densa, consisting of closely packed cells, forms a portion of the wall of the distal convoluted tubule adjacent to the vascular pole of the renal corpuscle.

Figure 14.7   ×125

Figure 14.7. Cortex, Kidney, Horse. Portions of three renal corpuscles, each with an accompanying macula densa, are present. In the horse the macula densa commonly consists of a stratified layer of cells.

Figure 14.8. Cortex, Kidney, Horse. A collecting tubule with clearly defined cells and a smooth lining can be contrasted with proximal convoluted tubules whose cells possess a brush border of microvilli.

Figure 14.9. Cortex, Kidney, Pig. The junction of a proximal convoluted tubule with the capsule of a renal corpuscle is shown.

Figure 14.10. Afferent Arteriole, Kidney, Pig. An afferent arteriole, with juxtaglomerular cells, is entering a glomerulus. The juxtaglomerular cells are epithelioid. Note that a macula densa borders the afferent arteriole.

Figure 14.8   ×250

Figure 14.9   ×250

Figure 14.10   ×250

Figure 14.11   ×250

Figure 14.15   ×250

Figure 14.12   ×250

Figure 14.11. Afferent and Efferent Arterioles, Kidney, Pig. Junction of a glomerulus with an afferent arteriole. A macula densa parallels the afferent arteriole.

Figure 14.12. Pars Radiata, l.s., Cortex, Kidney, Horse. The component tubules of a medullary ray include collecting tubules, as well as thick descending and thick ascending portions of the loop of Henle.

Figure 14.13. Renal Papilla, Kidney, Dog. Papillary ducts open onto the tip of a renal papilla.

Figure 14.14. Medulla, Kidney, Dog. Nuclei of the cells lining the thin segment of Henle's loop are rounded; those of endothelial cells of the vasa recta are flattened and more darkly stained.

Figure 14.15. Medulla, Kidney, Horse. Various portions of uriniferous tubules appear in transverse section.

Figure 14.13   ×12.5

Figure 14.14   ×250

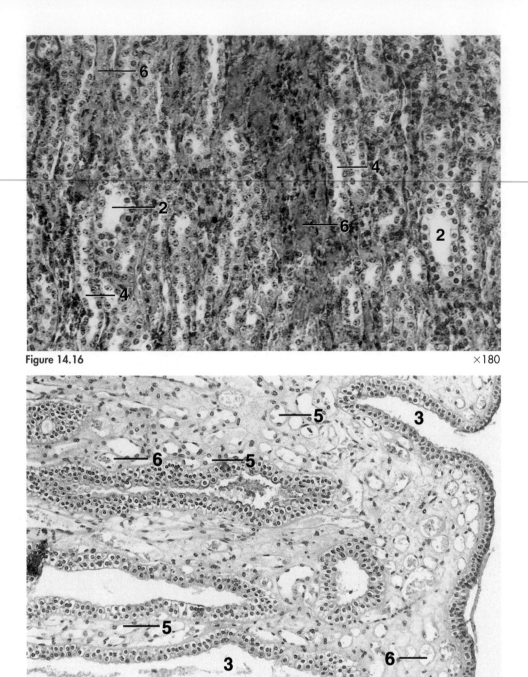

Figure 14.16   ×180

Figure 14.17   ×90

KEY	
1. Cavity of renal pelvis	4. Thick ascending, Henle's loop
2. Collecting tubule	5. Thin segment, Henle's loop
3. Papillary duct	6. Vasa recta

Figure 14.16. Medulla, Kidney, Cow (Trichrome). Longitudinal sections of vasa rectae and portions of uriniferous tubules. The vasa rectae are filled with red blood cells *(stained orange).*

Figure 14.17. Renal Papilla, Kidney, Goat. Papillary ducts near the tip of a renal papilla are lined by transitional epithelium.

Figure 14.18 ×250

Figure 14.18. Medulla, Kidney, Goat. A papillary duct, l.s., some distance away from the apex of the papilla, is lined by columnar cells. A thin segment of Henle's loop parallels the duct.

Figure 14.19. Medulla, Kidney, Goat (Silver). The collecting tubules are encircled by reticular fibers *(stained black)*. The fibers provide a supportive framework for other portions of the uriniferous tubules as well.

Figure 14.20. Urachus, Umbilical Cord, Cow. The urachus (allantoic stalk) is lined by a transitional epithelium. A portion of the lining is shown.

Figure 14.21. Ureter, x.s., Cat (Masson's). The middle circular layer of smooth muscle of the muscularis is most evident. Inner and outer longitudinal layers are present but sparse in this section.

Figure 14.19 ×250

Figure 14.20 ×125

Figure 14.21 ×62.5

Figure 14.22   ×25

Figure 14.26   ×250

KEY		
1. Capillary	5. Muscularis mucosae	
2. Lamina propria	6. Submucosa	
3. Mucous gland	7. Transitional epithelium	
4. Muscularis		

Figure 14.22. Ureter, x.s., Horse (Masson's). The proximal (anterior) portion of the horse's ureter contains tubuloalveolar mucous glands.

Figure 14.23. Ureter, x.s., Horse. Distally (posteriorly), the horse's ureter lacks mucous glands. The muscularis consists of an inner longitudinal, middle circular, and outer longitudinal layer of smooth muscle.

Figure 14.24. Urinary Bladder, Pig. The mucosa to a portion of the muscularis is shown. Scattered muscle cells of the muscularis mucosae are located adjacent to the lamina propria.

Figure 14.25. Urinary Bladder, Cow. The bladder contains a muscularis mucosae between the lamina propria and submucosa. Only a portion of the thick muscularis is shown.

Figure 14.26. Urinary Bladder, Goat. Numerous capillaries are located beneath the transitional epithelial lining of the bladder of ruminants.

Figure 14.23   ×12.5

Figure 14.24   ×125

Figure 14.25   ×12.5

Figure 14.29 ×125

KEY	
1. Cortex	5. Proximal convoluted tubule
2. Distal convoluted tubule	6. Renal corpuscle, large
3. Intralobular vein	7. Renal corpuscle, small
4. Medullary cone	

Figure 14.27. Kidney, Chicken. Cortical parenchyma and portion of a medullary cone are shown. An intralobular vein and both cortical (small) and medullary (large) renal corpuscles are apparent.

Figure 14.28. Kidney, Chicken. A portion of a medullary cone is surrounded by cortical lobules. The intralobular veins of two cortical lobules are clearly represented.

Figure 14.29. Cortex, Kidney, Chicken. An intralobular vein is surrounded by cortical tissue. Distal convoluted tubules are located mainly in the region of the intralobular vein.

Figure 14.27 ×36

Figure 14.28 ×36

Figure 14.30   ×360

Figure 14.32   ×90

Figure 14.31   ×250

KEY	
1. Collecting duct	9. Muscularis, outer layer
2. Collecting tubule	10. Proximal convoluted tubule
3. Distal convoluted tubule	11. Pseudostratified epithelium
4. Erythrocytes	12. Serosa
5. Glomerular epithelium	13. Thick ascending, Henle's loop
6. Lymphatic tissue	14. Thin segment, Henle's loop
7. Mesangial cells	15. Urinary space
8. Muscularis, inner layer	

Figure 14.30. Cortex, Kidney, Chicken. In the chicken the glomerular epithelium is composed of podocytes that have large, round or oval nuclei. The center of the glomerulus contains a compact mass of mesangial cells.

Figure 14.31. Medullary Cone, Kidney, Chicken. Various portions of uriniferous tubules (medullary type) are evident. Cells lining the thick ascending portions of Henle's loop show characteristic clear cytoplasmic blebs. A small portion of the cortex containing a proximal convoluted tubule can be seen on the upper right side.

Figure 14.32. Ureter, x.s., Chicken. The lamina propria is infiltrated with lymphocytes. Outer circular and inner longitudinal layers of the muscularis are distinguishable. The epithelium is pseudostratified columnar.

15

RESPIRATORY SYSTEM

MAMMALS

Air flows from the nostrils through a system of passages to the respiratory surfaces of the lungs. As it progresses, it becomes warmed, humidified, and cleansed of some of its particulate matter. Dust, which finds its way to the alveoli, is ultimately consumed by macrophages patrolling the tiny cul-de-sacs. The major components of the air-passage system are the **nasal cavity, pharynx, larynx, trachea, bronchi,** and the various smaller subdivisions of the bronchial tree leading to the alveoli.

Air from the naris enters the **vestibule,** the first part of the nasal cavity. The vestibule is lined by a stratified squamous epithelium, which is continuous with the skin externally and with the respiratory portion of the nasal cavity internally. In the horse hairy skin continues into the vestibule. A lamina propria and underlying submucosa support the vestibular epithelium.

The **respiratory portion** of the nasal cavity is lined by a ciliated, pseudostratified columnar epithelium with goblet cells. The lamina propria contains tubuloalveolar glands. The latter are mainly serous, but mucous and mixed glands do occur. Glands are sparse in carnivores. A submucosa supports the lamina propria.

The **olfactory epithelium** (pseudostratified columnar) is composed of olfactory (sensory) cells, supporting cells, and basal cells. Bowman's glands, tubular and mucoserous, occur within the lamina propria. They open to the surface through ducts lined by cuboidal or flattened cells. A submucosa lies below the lamina propria.

The **nasopharynx** and **oropharynx** are subdivisions of the pharynx. The former is lined by a ciliated, pseudostratified columnar epithelium with goblet cells, whereas the latter is covered by a stratified squamous epithelium. The lamina propria contains tubular mixed glands in the nasopharynx and mucous glands in the oropharynx. In carnivores the glands of the oropharynx are mixed. A network of elastic fibers separates the mucosa from an underlying sheet of skeletal muscle consisting of circularly and longitudinally arranged cells. The musculature is separated from an adventitia of loose connective tissue by a layer of connective tissue containing elastic networks.

The **larynx** is lined in part by a stratified squamous epithelium and partly by a ciliated, pseudostratified columnar epithelium. Numerous elastic fibers are present in the lamina propria. Glands (serous, mucous, and mixed) occur in the lamina propria and submucosa, but are lacking in the vocal and vestibular folds. Hyaline and elastic cartilage provide support for the laryngeal wall. The elastic cartilage of the **epiglottis** may be partially or completely replaced by adipose tissue, as in carnivores. Skeletal muscles are an integral part of the laryngeal structure.

The **trachea** is lined by a ciliated, pseudostratified columnar epithelium with goblet cells. A lamina propria and submucosa lie below the epithelium, but are not clearly demarcated from one another. Glands, mostly mixed, occur in the deeper layers of the lamina propria and within the submucosa. Rings of hyaline cartilage, which are incomplete dorsally, support the tracheal wall. A layer of smooth muscle, the **trachealis muscle,** is located dorsally in the trachea. It is positioned internal to the gap in the tracheal cartilages in the horse, pig, and ruminants. In the cat and dog it lies external to the gap. An adventitia of connective tissue completes the wall of the trachea.

The trachea bifurcates into bronchi, which enter the **lungs,** where they branch extensively. The lungs are covered by a **visceral pleura,** which is thick in large mammals and thinner in carnivores. Connective tissue and some smooth muscle form a part of the visceral pleura. The interior of the lungs contains a framework of connective tissue, rich in elastic fibers, which supports the bronchial tree and divides the lungs into lobules. The interlobular connective tissue is sparse in carnivores.

A ciliated, pseudostratified columnar epithelium with goblet cells lines the **bronchi.** The epithelium becomes reduced in height as the caliber of the bronchi diminishes. The lamina propria is surrounded by a layer of obliquely arranged smooth muscle. The connective tissue external to the musculature contains mixed glands and plates of hyaline cartilage. In the cat the bronchial cartilages may contain elastic fibers. When seen in histologic sections, the mucosa of large bronchi has few folds. Folds increase as the bronchi decrease in diameter.

The smallest bronchi give rise to suborders of **bronchioles.** The smallest of the latter, the terminal bronchioles, branch into two or more respiratory bronchioles, which divide into alveolar ducts that, in turn, empty into alveolar sacs.

Bronchioles lack cartilage and glands. Glands, however, may extend into bronchioles from bronchi in cats. Spirally or obliquely arranged smooth muscle forms part of the wall of a bronchiole. The amount of smooth muscle is proportional to the size of the bronchiole. Large bronchioles are lined by ciliated columnar cells, whereas the smallest (terminal) bronchioles are lined proximally by ciliated cuboidal cells and, distally, by nonciliated cells. The mucosa of the bronchioles is folded, unless the lungs were inflated at the time when the tissue was processed.

Respiratory bronchioles branch from the ends of terminal bronchioles. They are lined by a cuboidal epithelium, which becomes flattened distally, and their wall contains some smooth muscle. Alveoli are scattered within the epithelium. Respiratory bronchioles are best developed in the cat and dog.

Alveolar ducts branch from respiratory bronchioles. Their thin walls are constructed entirely of alveoli. The lip of each alveolus of an alveolar duct contains smooth muscle arranged circumferentially. The presence of the muscle gives the lip of the alveolus a knoblike appearance when histologic sections occur at right angles to the long axis of the muscle cells.

Ultimately, each alveolar duct branches into three or more **alveolar sacs.** No smooth muscle is present in the sacs. Therefore, the alveoli, which form the walls of the sacs, do not have lips with knoblike expansions as do those of the alveolar ducts.

Alveoli are lined mainly by exceedingly thin squamous epithelial cells (type I cells). Alveoli are separated from one another by a thin, highly vascularized layer of fine collagenous and elastic fibers. This layer, together with the squamous cells lining the adjacent alveoli, forms an alveolar septum.

CHICKEN

The nostrils, nasal cavity, pharynx, trachea, syrinx, bronchi, air capillaries, and air sacs comprise the respiratory system of the bird. The skin enters the nostrils to the first part of the nasal cavity, the **vestibule,** which is lined by a modified, keratinized, stratified squamous epithelium. It is characterized by epithelial cells that are organized into columns, giving the surface a wavy appearance. The **respiratory region** of the nasal cavity is lined by a ciliated, pseudostratified columnar epithelium. Mucous glands occur within the respiratory epithelium. The **olfactory epithelium** is pseudostratified columnar. It is located in the upper portions of the respiratory regions. Its structure, like that of mammals, is composed of basal, sensory, and supporting cells. Bowman's glands are present.

The **pharynx** is lined by a stratified squamous epithelium. A dense lamina propria and less dense submucosa lie below the epithelium. Salivary glands (mucous) occur within the lamina propria or submucosa. Bundles of skeletal muscle occur below the floor of the pharynx.

At the anterior end of the trachea is a cranial larynx, which is reinforced by a cartilaginous ring. A caudal larynx (syrinx) is located at the posterior end of the trachea. The **trachea** is supported by overlapping, complete cartilaginous rings. It is lined by a ciliated, pseudostratified columnar epithelium containing numerous, simple alveolar mucous glands. In the posterior portion of the trachea, the glands are replaced by goblet cells. A lamina propria and submucosa are present. Each consists of dense connective tissue. The submucosa is rich in elastic fibers.

The **syrinx,** or voice box, is located in the thoracic cavity at the point of tracheal bifurcation into two bronchi. Internal and external **tympanic membranes,** located in the region of the tracheal bifurcation, characterize the wall of the syrinx. **Intersyringeal cartilages** and a bony wedge, the **pessulus,** provide support in the region of the syrinx.

Each **extrapulmonary primary bronchus** enters a lung as an **intrapulmonary primary bronchus** (mesobronchus). **Secondary bronchi stem** from the primary bronchi and branch into numerous **parabronchi** (tertiary bronchi) within the lung. The latter anastomose with each other. Tiny, respiratory **air capillaries** form extensive networks interconnecting the tertiary bronchi.

Primary bronchi are lined by a ciliated pseudostratified columnar epithelium with mucous glands and goblet cells. Extrapulmonary primary bronchi have C-shaped cartilages, while the walls of intrapulmonary primary bronchi contain cartilaginous plates, which become scarce distally. Bundles of smooth muscle, mainly circular, occur below the lamina propria. Numerous elastic fibers are found throughout the connective tissue of the bronchi.

Secondary bronchi are lined by a ciliated, columnar epithelium with mucous cells. There is a lamina propria and a well-developed muscularis.

Parabronchi are lined by a cuboidal epithelium. A thin layer of connective tissue lies below the epithelium. Bundles of smooth muscle cells lie below the connective tissue layer. The inner wall of each tertiary bronchus is pierced by numerous openings, each of which leads into a cavity called an **atrium** (air vesicle). Atria are lined by a squamous to cuboidal epithelium. **Air capillaries,** lined by squamous cells, open into atria. Their simple squamous lining is a respiratory surface and is analogous to the lining epithelium of the alveoli of the mammalian lung. Numerous vascular capillaries surround the air capillaries and are separated from the latter by a basement membrane.

Air sacs are paired or unpaired, thin-walled structures occurring in the cervical, clavicular, thoracic, and abdominal regions of the body. They connect to the lungs by bronchi. Many of the hollow bones of the fowl contain extensions of the air sacs. Among others, these bones include the sternum, humerus, pelvic girdle, and most of the thoracic and cervical vertebrae. The air sacs are lined by squamous, ciliated cuboidal, and ciliated columnar cells. The epithelium is supported by a thin layer of connective tissue consisting of collagenous and elastic fibers. The sacs are poorly vascularized and do not participate in gas exchange.

Figure 15.1   ×12.5

Figure 15.4   ×125

Figure 15.2   ×12.5

KEY	
1. Basal cells	8. Olfactory cells, nuclei
2. Bone	9. Pseudostratified epithelium
3. Bowman's gland	10. Sensory hairs
4. Cartilage	11. Serous gland
5. Cavernous vein	12. Stratified squamous epithelium
6. Goblet cell	13. Supporting cells, nuclei
7. Nasal cavity	

Figure 15.1. Nasal Cavity, Vestibule, Dog. This portion of the vestibule is supported by hyaline cartilage and lined by a stratified squamous epithelium. Numerous cavernous veins occur throughout the connective tissue of the mucosa. In addition, there are tubular serous glands within the connective tissue.

Figure 15.2. Portion of Nasal Concha, Dog. The scroll-like nasal conchae are supported by spongy bone and are covered by a mucous membrane with a ciliated, pseudostratified columnar epithelium.

Figure 15.3. Olfactory Epithelium, Nasal Cavity, Dog (Masson's). This thick, pseudostratified columnar epithelium is composed of three types of cells. Basal cells are located at the level of the basement membrane. The nuclei of olfactory cells form a broad band in the central portion of the epithelium. The nuclei of supporting cells are pale and form the uppermost level of nuclei. The apices of olfactory cells bear sensory hairs.

Figure 15.4. Respiratory Epithelium, Nasal Concha, Dog. Ciliated, pseudostratified columnar epithelium with goblet cells and underlying, vascular, loose connective tissue and bone.

Figure 15.3   ×180

Figure 15.5 ×250

Figure 15.9 ×250

Figure 15.6 ×62.5

Figure 15.10 ×12.5

KEY	
1. Adipose tissue	9. Serous acinus
2. Arytenoid cartilage	10. Skeletal muscle
3. Duct	11. Stratified squamous
4. Elastic cartilage	epithelium, nonkeratinized
5. Intercalated duct	12. Striated duct
6. Lamina propria	13. Submucosa
7. Mixed gland	14. Taste bud
8. Pseudostratified epithelium	

Figure 15.7 ×25

Figure 15.5. Lateral Nasal Gland, Dog (Masson's). This serous gland is located in the maxillary sinus in carnivores.

Figure 15.6. Nasopharynx, Dog. This portion of the pharynx is lined by a ciliated, pseudostratified columnar epithelium with goblet cells. Mixed glands are present. The muscularis consists of skeletal muscle.

Figure 15.7. Epiglottis, Dog. The supporting elastic cartilage of the epiglottis is heavily infiltrated in its mid-region by adipose tissue in carnivores.

Figure 15.8. Epiglottis, l.s., Sheep. Blocklike chunks of elastic cartilage, without infiltrating adipose tissue, are found in the epiglottis of the sheep and goat.

Figure 15.9. Epiglottis, Sheep. Occasionally, taste buds are found in the epithelium of the laryngeal surface of the epiglottis.

Figure 15.10. Glottis, x.s., Goat. The glottis is supported by the arytenoid cartilages (elastic) and is lined by a nonkeratinized stratified squamous epithelium.

Figure 15.8 ×12.5

Figure 15.11   ×12.5

Figure 15.12   ×25

Figure 15.13   ×12.5

Figure 15.14   ×250

Figure 15.15   ×62.5

KEY	
1. Adipose tissue	10. Plasma cell
2. Arytenoid cartilage	11. Pseudostratified epithelium
3. Elastic fibers	12. Serous gland
4. Esophagus	13. Skeletal muscle
5. Goblet cell	14. Stratified squamous epithelium
6. Hyaline cartilage	15. Submucosa
7. Lamina propria	16. Trachea
8. Mixed gland	17. Trachealis muscle
9. Muscularis externa	18. Vocal ligament

Figure 15.11. Vocal Fold, l.s., Cat. Junction of the vocal fold with the arytenoid cartilage.

Figure 15.12. Vocal Fold, Goat (Orcein). The vocal fold consists of a fold of the mucous membrane. The vocal fold encloses the vocal ligament, which is a band of elastic fibers.

Figure 15.13. Trachea and Esophagus, x.s., Cat. Note that the trachealis muscle (smooth) lies external to the gap in the C-shaped cartilage in carnivores.

Figure 15.14. Trachea, x.s., Cat. The trachea is lined by a ciliated, pseudostratified columnar epithelium with goblet cells. The lamina propria contains a band of longitudinally oriented elastic fibers.

Figure 15.15. Trachea, x.s., Horse. A thick band of longitudinally arranged elastic fibers extends from the lamina propria into the submucosa.

Figure 15.16 ×25

Figure 15.20 ×25

KEY	
1. Adipose tissue	7. Mixed glands
2. Elastic fibers	8. Muscularis
3. Fibroelastic membrane	9. Perichondrium
4. Goblet cell	10. Pseudostratified epithelium
5. Hyaline cartilage	11. Tracheal glands
6. Lamina propria	12. Trachealis muscle

Figure 15.17 ×250

Figure 15.16. Trachea, x.s., Cow. In noncarnivores the trachealis muscle attaches to the perichondrium on the inside of the tracheal cartilage. The lamina propria and submucosa are both very rich in elastic fibers.

Figure 15.17. Trachea, x.s., Cow. The trachea is lined by a ciliated, pseudostratified columnar epithelium with goblet cells.

Figure 15.18. Trachea, x.s., Sheep (Orcein). A fibroelastic membrane surrounds the C-shaped tracheal cartilage and also spans the gap in the cartilage.

Figure 15.19. Trachea, x.s., Goat (Orcein). Numerous elastic fibers occur below the epithelium. Elastic fibers are also present where the trachealis muscle joins with the perichondrium.

Figure 15.20. Primary Bronchus, Extrapulmonary, x.s., Dog (Mallory's). Plates of hyaline cartilage support the wall of the bronchus. Smooth muscle bundles of the muscularis occur between the plates and internal to them.

Figure 15.18 ×12.5

Figure 15.19 ×25

Figure 15.21   ×25

Figure 15.25   ×250

Figure 15.22   ×62.5

KEY	
1. Alveolus	7. Lamina propria
2. Bronchiole	8. Lymphatic nodule
3. Columnar epithelium, ciliated	9. Mixed gland
4. Elastic band	10. Muscularis
5. Goblet cell	11. Pseudostratified epithelium
6. Hyaline cartilage	12. Serous gland

Figure 15.21. Bronchus, x.s., Cow (Masson's).

Figure 15.22. Bronchus, x.s., Cow. Detail of the wall of a bronchus. Numerous lymphocytes are present below the epithelium.

Figure 15.23. Small Bronchus, x.s., and Bronchioles, Cat. Bronchioles lack cartilaginous plates and possess a simple epithelium.

Figure 15.24. Large Bronchiole, x.s., Cat. In cats submucosal serous glands extend from bronchi into the bronchioles.

Figure 15.25. Large Bronchiole, x.s., Cat. Detail of a portion of the bronchiole shown in Figure 15.24.

Figure 15.23   ×25

Figure 15.24   ×62.5

Figure 15.26   ×125

Figure 15.27   ×125

Figure 15.28   ×125

Figure 15.29   ×62.5

Figure 15.30   ×125

KEY	
1. Alveolar duct	6. Elastic fibers
2. Alveolar sac	7. Macrophage
3. Alveolus	8. Muscularis
4. Bronchiole	9. Respiratory bronchiole
5. Cuboidal epithelium	10. Smooth muscle

Figure 15.26. Bronchioles, Pig (Orcein). The tissues of the lung are heavily infiltrated with elastic fibers.

Figure 15.27. Respiratory Bronchiole, x.s., Cat. Respiratory bronchioles are lined by a cuboidal epithelium and have alveoli in their walls.

Figure 15.28. Respiratory Bronchiole, l.s., Sheep.

Figure 15.29. Alveolar Ducts and Alveolar Sacs, Sheep. An alveolar duct is characterized by the presence of smooth muscle arranged circumferentially in the lips of the alveoli that form its wall. Conversely, the alveoli of alveolar sacs lack smooth muscle.

Figure 15.30. Alveolar Duct, x.s., Sheep. Detail of an alveolar duct. The smooth muscle associated with the entrance of the alveoli that form the wall of the duct is evident.

Figure 15.31 ×360

Figure 15.34 ×12.5

KEY	
1. Alveolar septum	7. Macrophage
2. Alveolus	8. Mesothelium
3. Bronchiole	9. Septum
4. Bronchus	10. Type II alveolar cell
5. Elastic band	11. Visceral pleura
6. Erythrocyte in capillary	

Figure 15.31. Alveoli, Cat. Detail of alveolar septa.

Figure 15.32. Visceral Pleura, Dog. The visceral pleura of carnivores is relatively thin.

Figure 15.33. Visceral Pleura, Horse. The visceral pleura of domestic mammals, except carnivores, is thick. Incomplete septa extend inward from the visceral pleura in the horse.

Figure 15.34. Visceral Pleura, Pig. Lungs are highly lobulated in the pig and ruminants. Unlike those of the horse, the septa are complete.

Figure 15.32 ×250

Figure 15.33 ×25

Figure 15.35

×62.5

Figure 15.39

×125

Figure 15.36

×125

KEY	
1. Alveolus	9. Parietal pleura
2. Basal cells	10. Pseudostratified epithelium
3. Epidermis	11. Pulmonary vein
4. Intercostal muscle	12. Pyknotic nucleus
5. Lamina propria	13. Septum
6. Mucous gland	14. Smooth muscle
7. Nerve	15. Turbinate cartilage
8. Neuromuscular spindle	16. Vestibular epithelium

Figure 15.35. Parietal Pleura, Cat. Parietal pleura and intercostal muscle. The parietal pleura lines the wall of the pleural cavity. It consists of a mesothelium and underlying connective tissue.

Figure 15.36. Lung, Cow (Masson's). In the cow and pig, pulmonary veins have thick bands of circularly arranged smooth muscle.

Figure 15.37. Nasal Cavity, Chicken. The vestibule is lined by a uniquely structured, keratinized, stratified squamous epithelium (see Fig. 15.38). The vestibular epithelium blends with the epidermis on the inner side of each nostril. In this micrograph these epithelia lie to either side of a turbinate cartilage.

Figure 15.38. Vestibular Epithelium, Chicken. This keratinized, stratified squamous epithelium is characterized by the presence of columns of cells. The uppermost cells in each column have pyknotic nuclei. One or two layers of basal cells are present. The outer surface of the epithelium presents a corrugated appearance.

Figure 15.39. Respiratory Epithelium, Chicken (Masson's). This ciliated, pseudostratified columnar epithelium is interrupted by simple, branched, alveolar mucous glands.

Figure 15.37

×62.5

Figure 15.38

×250

Figure 15.40 ×250

Figure 15.41 ×12.5

Figure 15.42 ×62.5

Figure 15.43 ×125

Figure 15.44 ×25

KEY	
1. Basal cell	7. Olfactory cells, nuclei
2. Bony tracheal ring	8. Pseudostratified epithelium
3. Bowman's gland	9. Skeletal muscle
4. Cartilaginous tracheal ring	10. Stratified squamous
5. Mucous gland	epithelium
6. Nerve	11. Supporting cell, nucleus

Figure 15.40. Olfactory Epithelium, Chicken (Masson's). This pseudostratified columnar epithelium is similar to that found in mammals (see Fig. 15.3). It is composed of basal, olfactory, and supporting cells.

Figure 15.41. Trachea, l.s., Chicken. Cartilaginous tracheal rings are complete and overlap each other. When the trachea is cut longitudinally, as in this preparation, the rings are cut transversely and present a lenticular profile.

Figure 15.42. Trachea, x.s., Chicken. Simple alveolar mucous glands occur in the ciliated, pseudostratified columnar epithelium. Portions of two overlapping tracheal rings are present. The inner ring was cut through its thin edge, while the outer one was cut through its thick middle region (see Fig. 15.41 for an example of the shape of a tracheal ring that has been cut transversely).

Figure 15.43. Trachea, x.s., Chicken. Intraepithelial mucous glands are abundant in the trachea of the chicken (also see Fig. 15.39).

Figure 15.44. Trachea, Near Syrinx, Chicken. The majority of the posterior, complete rings of the trachea shown here are bony. The ciliated pseudostratified columnar epithelium of the trachea is followed in the syrinx by a stratified squamous epithelium.

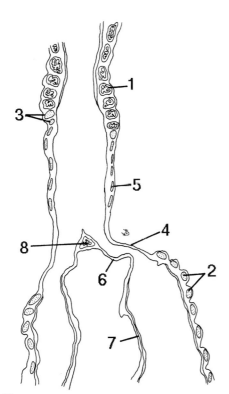

Figure 15.45

KEY	
1. Bony tracheal ring	6. Internal tympanic
2. Bronchial rings	membrane
3. Cartilaginous tracheal rings	7. Medial bronchial wall
4. External tympanic membrane	8. Pessulus
5. Intermediate syringeal	9. Stratified squamous
cartilage	epithelium

Figure 15.45. Trachea, Syrinx and Primary Bronchi, l.s., Chicken.

Figure 15.46. Syrinx, l.s., Chicken.

Figure 15.47. Syrinx, l.s., Chicken. A portion of the external tympanic membrane and intermediate syringeal cartilage.

Figure 15.46   ×25

Figure 15.47   ×125

Figure 15.48 ×62.5

Figure 15.48. Syrinx, l.s., Chicken (Orcein). Intermediate syringeal cartilages are connected by numerous elastic fibers.

Figure 15.49. Syrinx, l.s.,Chicken. Portion of pessulus and internal tympanic membrane. The latter is covered by both a ciliated, stratified columnar epithelium and by a stratified squamous epithelium.

Figure 15.50. Tympanic Membrane and Primary Bronchus, Chicken. Three transected bronchial cartilages. Bronchial cartilages are incomplete (C-shaped). They do not extend to the medial side of the bronchus.

Figure 15.51. Lung, Chicken. Longitudinal section through a secondary bronchus and parabronchi. The presence of numerous cup-shaped atria in the parabronchus distinguish this part of the bronchial tree from the secondary bronchus.

Figure 15.49 ×125

Figure 15.50 ×12.5

Figure 15.51 ×25

Figure 15.52

×62.5

Figure 15.53

×250

Figure 15.54

×250

Figure 15.55

×125

Figure 15.52. Lung, Chicken. Cross section of a parabronchus and a portion of an adjacent secondary bronchus.

Figure 15.53. Lung, Chicken. Detail of the wall of a parabronchus. Note the continuity of the air capillaries with the atria. The latter are lined by an epithelium that varies from simple cuboidal to simple squamous.

Figure 15.54. Abdominal Air Sac, Chicken. The wall of the air sac consists of a connective tissue lamina and an epithelium that may be simple squamous, cuboidal, or ciliated columnar. Air sacs are not well vascularized.

Figure 15.55. Humerus, x.s., Chicken (Masson's). Many bones of the chicken contain extensions of air sacs.

16

ENDOCRINE SYSTEM

MAMMALS

The pituitary, pineal, thyroid, parathyroid, and adrenal glands possess certain features that distinguish them as organs of the endocrine system. They are very rich in wide, thin-walled vessels called sinusoids. The sinusoids are intimately associated with parenchymal cells, whose secretory products (hormones) pass directly into the circulatory system. Endocrine glands lack ducts. In contrast, exocrine glands convey their secretions (e.g., enzymes, mucus, and bile) through ducts to a mucosal or skin surface.

Endocrine cells are not limited to the glands presented in this chapter. For example, hormones are secreted by interstitial cells of the testes, corpora lutea and ovarian follicles, islets of Langerhans, and enterochromaffin cells of the gastrointestinal epithelium.

The **pituitary gland** (hypophysis) is a major endocrine gland that is suspended from the hypothalamus of the brain. It releases several hormones, many of which influence the activity of other endocrine glands. The glandular portion, the **adenohypophysis,** forms from an outpocketing of the ectoderm of the dorsal portion of the oral cavity, called Rathke's pouch. The pars distalis, pars tuberalis, and pars intermedia constitute the adenohypophysis. The neural part of the pituitary gland, the **neurohypophysis,** is derived from a ventral outpocketing of the diencephalon. It is divisible into a median eminence, infundibular stalk, and pars nervosa.

The **pars distalis** is the largest portion of the pituitary gland. The parenchyma consists of irregular cords of cells separated by sinusoids and sparse connective tissue. There are two main types of parenchymal cells: **chromophobes,** characterized by a small amount of cytoplasm that stains poorly, and **chromophils,** with more abundant cytoplasm that is readily stained. The chromophils are classified as **acidophils** (alpha cells) and **basophils** (beta cells). Basophils tend to be larger than acidophils. Chromophobes are smaller than chromophils and are most evident in groups, appearing as clusters of closely packed nuclei in tissue sections.

The **pars intermedia** is situated between the pars distalis and the pars nervosa. In the horse these regions are closely apposed. In other domestic mammals the pars intermedia and pars distalis are partially separated by a small cleft, the **hypophyseal cavity,** which is the **vestigial cavity of Rathke's pouch.** The pars intermedia consists predominantly of basophilic cells. Follicles filled with colloid are often present.

The **pars tuberalis** is mainly located around the infundibular stalk. It is composed primarily of cords, clusters, and follicles of small, faintly basophilic cells.

The neurohypophysis contains numerous unmyelinated nerve fibers whose cell bodies are located in the supraoptic and paraventricular nuclei of the hypothalamus. Their axons converge at the **median eminence** (ventral boundary of the third ventricle) and form the hypothalamohypophyseal tract. They pass through the narrow **infundibular stalk** to the **pars nervosa** (infundibular process). The neurosecretions of these cells move along within the axons and accumulate at the terminal regions of the nerve fibers as **Herring bodies,** which are best demonstrated with special staining methods. Overall, the pars nervosa has an unorganized, fibrous appearance, and individual axons are indistinct. Numerous **pituicytes** (neuroglial cells) are scattered among the nerve fibers. They possess round to oval nuclei and long cytoplasmic processes. Their cytoplasm cannot be distinguished from nerve fibers in routine histologic preparations.

The **infundibular cavity,** which is continuous with the third ventricle and lined by ependymal cells, extends deep into the pars nervosa in the cat and pig and to a lesser extent in the dog and horse. In ruminants the cavity does not reach beyond the infundibular stalk. These relationships are evident in midsagittal sections of the pituitary gland.

The **pineal gland** (pineal body; epiphysis cerebri) is a dorsal evagination of the roof of the diencephalon. It is covered by connective tissue of the pia mater and divided into lobules by septa of connective tissue. The parenchyma is composed predominantly of **pinealocytes,** which are arranged as clusters, cords, or follicles. These epithelioid cells have a round nucleus and acidophilic cytoplasm. Neuroglial cells are also present.

Each lobe of the **thyroid gland** is surrounded by a thin capsule of connective tissue and divided into lobules by thin trabeculae. The latter are continuous with sparse intralobular connective tissue that contains numerous sinusoids. In the pig and cow the connective tissue is abundant. Each lobule consists of numerous **follicles** of various sizes that are frequently filled with colloid. The follicular cells vary in height, depending on the state of activity of the follicle. Their appearance changes from squamous or low cuboidal in the resting stage to cuboidal or columnar in the active stage. In an active follicle the periphery of the colloid adjacent to the apical surface of the follicular cells is vacuolated. In an inactive follicle, the colloid has a smoother peripheral surface and vacuoles are not present.

Parafollicular (C) cells occur among the cells that line the thyroid follicles and also between the follicles. They are larger and have a paler cytoplasm than the follicular cells. Their nuclei are relatively large and pale. Parafollicular cells usually occur singly, but may also appear in groups. In the dog these cells are particularly abundant.

The **parathyroid glands** are classified as internal and external. Those that are adjacent to or embedded in the thyroid gland are the internal parathyroids. The external parathyroids lie a variable distance away from the thyroid gland. The parathyroid glands are surrounded by a thin capsule of connective tissue, which may be absent where the glands are deeply embedded within the thyroid gland. A stroma of connective tissue is well developed in the pig and cow, but is sparse in other domestic mammals.

The parenchyma of the parathyroid gland consists primarily of clusters and cords of **principal** (chief) **cells.** There are two different functional stages of the principal cell. The **light principal cell** is inactive and has a large, pale nucleus and pale, acidophilic cytoplasm. The **dark principal cell** is a smaller, active cell with a small, dark nucleus and a deeply acidophilic cytoplasm. In the sheep and goat, light cells tend to be located peripheral to the more central, dark cells. In the other domestic mammals these cells are distributed randomly.

Oxyphilic cells are large cells with an acidophilic cytoplasm and a pyknotic nucleus. They have been reported to occur in small numbers in the parathyroid glands of the horse and cow, particularly older animals.

The paired **adrenal glands** are situated close to the anterior end of the kidneys. The glands are covered by a capsule of dense irregular connective tissue that sometimes contains smooth muscle. Clusters of epithelioid cortical cells also occur in the capsule. Thin trabeculae project partially into the parenchyma.

Each adrenal gland is organized into a peripheral cortex and a central medulla. The **adrenal cortex** is divided into four zones. The **zona glomerulosa** (zone multiformis) is the outermost zone. In the carnivore, horse, and pig the parenchymal cells of this region are columnar and arranged into arcs. In the horse the columnar cells are especially tall. In ruminants the zona glomerulosa contains polyhedral cells that form irregular clusters or cords.

The **zona intermedia** lies between the zone glomerulosa and the zona fasciculata. It consists of small, closely packed cells. This zone is seen more often in the horse and carnivore than in the other domestic mammals.

The **zona fasciculata,** the widest zone of the adrenal cortex, is formed by radially arranged cords of cuboidal or polyhedral cells. The cords are one or two cells thick and separated by sinusoids. The cytoplasm of the cells in this zone frequently appears foamy because of the presence of numerous lipid vacuoles.

The **zona reticularis** is the innermost zone of the adrenal cortex. It is arranged as an irregular network of anastomosing cords of cells surrounded by sinusoids.

The **adrenal medulla** is composed mostly of columnar or polyhedral chromaffin cells, which form clusters and anastomosing cords separated by sinusoids. In domestic mammals an outer and inner zone of the medulla can often be distinguished. The former consists of larger, more darkly stained cells, and the latter contains smaller, more lightly stained cells. Ganglion cells, either individually or in clusters, are scattered through the medulla. Because the cortex and medulla interdigitate at their junction, projections of the zona reticularis may appear within the medulla.

CHICKEN

As in mammals, the **pituitary gland** (hypophysis) of the chicken is attached to the base of the brain below the diencephalon and is encapsulated by the dura mater. The **adenohypophysis** is composed of the pars distalis and pars tuberalis. A pars intermedia is absent. The **pars distalis** is divided into a **cephalic region** and a **caudal region**. Both regions contain cords of acidophils and basophils, and clusters of chromophobes. The acidophils of the cephalic region are pale, and those of the caudal zone are more darkly stained. Thus, the cephalic zone appears more basophilic, and the caudal zone appears more acidophilic. The cords of cells of the former are more closely packed than those of the latter. Some parenchymal cells of the pars distalis may be arranged around a lumen filled with colloid, especially in older birds. Cysts lined by ciliated cells and mucous cells also occur in this part of the pituitary gland.

The **pars tuberalis** surrounds the infundibulum and spreads dorsally over the ventral surface of the brain for a short distance. Ventrally, it extends to the posterior margin of the cephalic zone of the pars distalis. The pars tuberalis contains small, round to elongated, slightly basophilic cells that are arranged in several layers.

The **neurohypophysis** includes the median eminence of the tuber cinereum, the infundibular stalk, and the pars nervosa (infundibular process). The **median eminence** and the **infundibular stalk** consist primarily of nerve fibers, neuroglial cells, and ependymal cells that line the infundibular cavity. The **pars nervosa** has an irregular surface and consists of numerous lobules. Each lobule contains a diverticulum of the infundibular cavity that is lined by ependymal cells. The latter are surrounded by irregular masses of tissue consisting of pituicytes and other neuroglial cells, nerve fibers, and Herring bodies.

The **pineal gland** (epiphysis cerebri) is a small, conical body that is situated between the cerebral hemispheres and the cerebellum. It is surrounded by connective tissue and is composed of a **body** and a narrow, ventral **stalk** that is attached to the roof of the third ventricle. The parenchyma of the gland is arranged into lobules separated by thin septa of connective tissue. The lobules contain cells, predominantly pinealocytes, that form rosettes or follicles.

The **thyroid glands** are composed of numerous colloid-filled follicles, as in mammals. Cells that are similar in function to the parafollicular cells of mammals, however, occur in the ultimobranchial bodies, rather than the thyroid glands, of the chicken.

The **parathyroid glands** are each surrounded by a capsule of connective tissue. The parenchyma is composed of irregular cords of chief cells, separated by connective tissue and numerous sinusoids.

The **adrenal glands** are enclosed within a capsule of dense connective tissue. Unlike mammals, the parenchyma is not organized into a distinct cortex and medulla. Instead, it is composed of intermingled **cortical** (interrenal) **tissue** and **medullary** (chromaffin) **tissue**. The cortical cells are arranged as irregular cords. These cells have dark nuclei and appear columnar when the cords are sectioned longitudinally. In a cross section of a cord the cells appear tall and pyramidal with several cells arranged radially. Medullary tissue is composed of polygonal cells. They are larger than cortical cells and possess a large, round nucleus and basophilic cytoplasm. Ganglion cells occur among the medullary cells. Two ganglia (the cranial and caudal suprarenal ganglia) are apposed to the surface of the adrenal glands and are frequently included in histologic sections of this gland.

Figure 16.1   ×18

Figure 16.2   ×62.5

Figure 16.3   ×62.5

KEY	
1. Cavity of Rathke's pouch	6. Median eminence
2. Ependymal cells	7. Pars distalis
3. Follicle	8. Pars intermedia
4. Infundibular cavity	9. Pars nervosa
5. Infundibular stalk	10. Pars tuberalis

Figure 16.1. Pituitary Gland, Cat. Parasagittal section showing all major components. In domestic mammals, except the horse, the cavity of Rathke's pouch persists in the adult. (Photomicrograph of a histologic section borrowed from the College of Veterinary Medicine, Iowa State University.)

Figure 16.2. Pituitary Gland, Cat. Detail of the Infundibular stalk and pars tuberalis. Note the presence of small follicles in the pars tuberalis lined by faintly basophilic epithelial cells. (Photomicrograph of a histologic section borrowed from the College of Veterinary Medicine, Iowa State University.)

Figure 16.3. Pituitary Gland, Cat. Pars intermedia, pars distalis, and pars nervosa. (Photomicrograph of a histologic section borrowed from the College of Veterinary Medicine, Iowa State University.)

Figure 16.4   ×125

Figure 16.4. Pituitary Gland, Dog. Detail of the pars distalis, pars intermedia, and pars nervosa.

Figure 16.5. Pituitary Gland, Parasagittal Section, Horse. Although present in other domestic animals, the cavity of Rathke's pouch is lacking in the horse.

Figure 16.6. Pituitary Gland, Horse (Alcian Blue, Orange G, Schiff's Reagent). Pars distalis, pars intermedia, and pars nervosa. Note the presence of follicles in the pars intermedia.

Figure 16.7. Pituitary Gland, Horse (Alcian Blue, Orange G, Schiff's Reagent). Detail of the pars intermedia and pars nervosa. The latter has a distinctive fibrous appearance.

Figure 16.5

Figure 16.6   ×12.5

Figure 16.7   ×125

Figure 16.8 ×250

Figure 16.10 ×25

KEY	
1. Acidophil	5. Infundibular stalk
2. Basophil	6. Pars distalis
3. Chromophobes	7. Pars tuberalis
4. Infundibular cavity	8. Sinusoid

Figure 16.8. Pituitary Gland, Horse (Alcian Blue, Orange G, Schiff's Reagent). Detail of the pars distalis. In this preparation acidophils are orange, whereas basophils vary from blue to red. Chromophobes are small and pale.

Figure 16.9. Pituitary Gland, Horse. Detail of the pars distalis. Chromophobes appear in clusters and have closely spaced nuclei.

Figure 16.10. Pituitary Gland, Horse. A portion of the infundibular stalk, pars distalis, and pars tuberalis.

Figure 16.9 ×180

Figure 16.11   ×25

Figure 16.12   ×125

Figure 16.13   ×25

Figure 16.14   ×125

Figure 16.15   ×250

KEY	
1. Adipose tissue	7. Parafollicular cell
2. Colloid	8. Parafollicular cells
3. Fibers of neuroglial cells	9. Parathyroid gland
4. Follicle	10. Pineal gland
5. Follicle, tangential cut	11. Pineal stalk
6. Follicular cell	12. Pinealocytes

Figure 16.11. Pineal Gland, Dog. This gland consists primarily of pinealocytes and is located in the midline of the epithalamus.

Figure 16.12. Pineal Gland, Dog. Detail of the gland.

Figure 16.13. Thyroid and Parathyroid Glands, Dog. The basophilic, highly cellular parathyroid gland contrasts with the numerous colloid-filled follicles of the thyroid gland.

Figure 16.14. Thyroid Gland, Inactive, Dog. Parafollicular cells (C-cells) have pale-staining cytoplasm. In the dog they are particularly numerous and frequently occur in groups.

Figure 16.15. Thyroid Gland, Inactive, Dog. Large, pale-staining parafollicular cells often form a part of the cellular lining of a thyroid follicle.

Figure 16.16   ×125

Figure 16.20   ×62.5

Figure 16.17   ×250

KEY	
1. Cilia	7. Follicular cell, pigmented
2. Colloid	8. Light cell
3. Cyst	9. Principal cells
4. Dark cell	10. Space artifact
5. Erythrocytes in sinusoid	11. Stroma
6. Follicular cell	

Figure 16.16. Thyroid Gland, Active, Horse. Active thyroid follicles are characterized by tall follicular cells and vacuolated colloid. Compare with Figures 16.15 and 16.17.

Figure 16.17. Thyroid Gland, Inactive, Goat. The high degree of vascularity of the thyroid gland is well illustrated in this micrograph. Pigment granules accumulate in the follicle cells of older animals.

Figure 16.18. Parathyroid Gland, Dog. Cysts containing colloid frequently occur in the parathyroid gland. Such cysts are lined by a ciliated columnar epithelium.

Figure 16.19. Parathyroid Gland, Dog. Both light and dark principal cells are visible. The active, dark cells have a nucleus with condensed chromatin and a dark, acidophilic cytoplasm. The inactive, light cells have a larger and paler nucleus and a lighter, acidophilic cytoplasm.

Figure 16.20. Parathyroid Gland, Cow. The stroma of connective tissue of the parathyroid gland of cows and pigs is abundant.

Figure 16.18   ×125

Figure 16.19   ×250

Figure 16.21   ×62.5

Figure 16.25   ×25

Figure 16.22   ×250

Figure 16.23   ×62.5

Figure 16.24   ×62.5

KEY	
1. Capsule	7. Sinusoid
2. Epithelioid cells	8. Zona fasciculata
3. Ganglion cell	9. Zona glomerulosa
4. Medulla	10. Zona intermedia
5. Medulla, inner region	11. Zona reticularis
6. Medulla, outer region	

Figure 16.21. Adrenal Gland, Dog. Adrenal cortex and capsule. The cells of the zona glomerulosa are arranged into arclike formations in carnivores, horses, and pigs.

Figure 16.22. Adrenal Gland, Cat. Detail of a portion of the cortex. A zona intermedia occurs between the zona glomerulosa and zona fasciculata. It is especially well developed in carnivores and horses. It consists of small, polyhedral cells. Cells of the zona fasciculata are characteristically highly vacuolated.

Figure 16.23. Adrenal Gland, Horse. Adrenal cortex and capsule. The zona glomerulosa consists of high arcs composed of especially tall epithelial cells in the horse. Clusters of epithelioid cortical cells frequently occur in the capsule of the adrenal gland. A distinct intermediate zone separates the zona glomerulosa from the zona fasciculata.

Figure 16.24. Adrenal Gland, Horse. An autonomic ganglion, surrounded by cells of the zona reticularis, is situated in the medulla.

Figure 16.25. Adrenal Gland, Cow. Portions of the cortex and medulla. The medulla is subdivided into an outer region of darkly stained cells and an inner portion of lightly stained cells.

Figure 16.26   ×62.5

Figure 16.27   ×125

Figure 16.28   ×250

Figure 16.29   ×12.5

Figure 16.30   ×250

KEY	
1. Capsule	12. Medulla, outer region
2. Chromaffin cells	13. Pars distalis, caudal
3. Chromophils	14. Pars distalis, cephalic
4. Chromophobes	15. Pars nervosa
5. Colloid	16. Pars tuberalis
6. Cyst	17. Sinusoid, with erythrocytes
7. Diencephalon	18. Skull
8. Ganglion cell	19. Zona fasciculata
9. Infundibular cavity	20. Zona glomerulosa
10. Infundibular stalk	21. Zona intermedia
11. Medulla, inner region	22. Zona reticularis

Figure 16.26. Adrenal Gland, Cow. Portion of the adrenal cortex. The cells of the zona glomerulosa are arranged into irregular groups and cords in ruminants. Compare with Figures 16.21, 16.22, and 16.23.

Figure 16.27. Adrenal Gland, Cow. The basophilic cells of the outer region of the adrenal medulla contrast with the paler cells of the inner region.

Figure 16.28. Adrenal Gland, Sheep (Masson's). Adrenal medulla with ganglion cells and cells of the zona reticularis amid the chromaffin cells.

Figure 16.29. Pituitary Gland, parasagittal section, Chicken. In the chicken the pars distalis is divisible into a cephalic zone and a caudal zone. The cephalic zone is more basophilic. Ciliated cysts commonly occur within the pars distalis (see Fig. 16.32 for detail of a cyst).

Figure 16.30. Pituitary Gland, Chicken. The cephalic zone of the pars distalis consists of closely packed cords of chromophils and chromophobes. Some cords have a lumen filled with colloid.

Figure 16.31 ×250

Figure 16.32 ×250

Figure 16.33 ×250

Figure 16.34 ×125

Figure 16.35 ×25

KEY	
1. Acidophil	8. Mucous cell
2. Basophil	9. Pars distalis, caudal
3. Capsule	10. Pars tuberalis
4. Cerebellum	11. Pineal gland
5. Ciliated cell	12. Pituicyte
6. Granulocytes	13. Sinusoid
7. Infundibular stalk	14. Skull

Figure 16.31. Pituitary Gland, Chicken. In the caudal zone of the pars distalis, the cells of the cords are more loosely arranged than those of the cephalic zone. Acidophils have a more intensely stained cytoplasm than those of the cephalic zone, and they can be readily distinguished from basophils.

Figure 16.32. Pituitary Gland, Chicken. Portion of a cyst, in the pars distalis, lined by ciliated cells and mucous cells.

Figure 16.33. Pituitary Gland, Chicken. Portions of the pars tuberalis and adjacent infundibular stalk. The cells of the pars tuberalis are rounded to elongated with a finely granular, slightly basophilic cytoplasm and a round to oval nucleus.

Figure 16.34. Pituitary Gland, Chicken. A group of pituicytes within the pars nervosa. Pituicytes have a clear cytoplasm and a large, vesicular nucleus.

Figure 16.35. Pineal Gland, parasagittal section, Chicken. The body of the pineal gland, portion of the overlying skull, and the cerebellum.

Figure 16.36 ×125

Figure 16.36. Pineal Gland, Chicken. The parenchymal cells of the pineal gland are arranged as compact masses (rosettes) or as round to oval follicles with distinct lumens.

Figure 16.37. Parathyroid Gland, Chicken. This gland consists of chief cells arranged into a feltwork of anastomosing cords. The cords are surrounded by strands of connective tissue and numerous sinusoids.

Figure 16.38. Adrenal Gland, Chicken. Cords of cortical cells are interwoven between clumps and irregular masses of medullary cells throughout the gland.

Figure 16.39. Adrenal Gland, Chicken. Detail of cortical and medullary cells. Cortical cells are columnar. When longitudinal cuts have been made through cords of cortical cells, the cells form a bilayer. When cords are cut transversely, the cells are seen to be arranged radially. Medullary cells are polygonal, are larger than cortical cells, and possess basophilic cytoplasm. They are arranged as clumps or irregular masses.

Figure 16.37 ×250

Figure 16.38 ×62.5

Figure 16.39 ×250

17

MALE REPRODUCTIVE SYSTEM

MAMMALS

The male reproductive system includes the testes, the system of ducts that leads from them, the penis, and accessory glands.

The **testes** are contained in the scrotum and are compound tubular glands that are invested by a thick capsule of dense irregular connective tissue, the **tunica albuginea**. This capsule is rich in smooth muscle in the stallion. The tunica albuginea is covered by a peritoneum, **the visceral layer of the tunica vaginalis**. The latter is composed of a mesothelium and underlying connective tissue that blends with that of the tunica albuginea. Septa of connective tissue extend from the tunica albuginea into the testis, partially or completely dividing the testis into lobules. These septa are thin in ruminants and thicker in the carnivore, stallion, and boar. Centrally, the septa may merge with the loose connective tissue of the **mediastinum testis**.

Within each lobule of the testis there are convoluted **seminiferous tubules**. They are lined by a stratified epithelium of **spermatogenic cells** and Sertoli cells. The spermatogenic cells give rise to **spermatozoa. Spermatogonia,** the most immature spermatogenic cells, are small, round cells with dark, round nuclei that lie adjacent to the basement membrane. These undergo mitotic divisions and produce **primary spermatocytes,** larger cells whose nuclei often show distinct chromatin. Primary spermatocytes undergo the first meiotic division, giving rise to smaller, **secondary spermatocytes.** Secondary spermatocytes are rarely observed because they undergo the second meiotic division shortly after they arise, forming haploid **spermatids.** Early spermatids are round cells with pale nuclei that occur in clusters toward the lumen of the seminiferous tubule. Late spermatids are characterized by small, oval to elongated, dark heads and long, faint tails that project into the lumen. They are eventually released from the seminiferous epithelium as spermatozoa.

Various combinations of developing spermatogenic cells occur within the epithelium of a seminiferous tubule. These cell associations (stages) are unique and occupy only a portion of the length of each tubule. The total number of different stages varies with different animals; for example, rats are known to have 14 different stages, while mice have 12 and pigs have eight.

The cell mix within each stage can be observed while examining a histologic section of the testis. In sections through some seminiferous tubules, for example, spermatogonia, two layers of primary spermatocytes, and numerous early spermatids may be apparent; in another segment there may be spermatogonia, a single layer of primary spermatocytes, and numerous early and late spermatids. Other spermatogenic cell combinations, characteristic of the animal, become apparent as more tubules are examined.

Sertoli cells are fewer in number than the spermatogenic cells. They are distinguished by a pale oval or triangular nucleus that has a prominent nucleolus and occasional cleftlike infoldings. They are tall cells that extend from the basement membrane to the lumen of the tubule, but their boundaries are indistinct in routine histologic preparations. Numerous lateral and apical invaginations of their cell membranes embrace the differentiating spermatogenic cells.

Flattened, contractile **myoid cells** lie just outside the basement membrane of each seminiferous tubule. The connective tissue between adjacent tubules contains polyhedral **interstitial** (Leydig) **cells**. These produce testosterone and are particularly abundant in the stallion and boar. They are recognized by their small, round nucleus and an acidophilic, often foamy cytoplasm.

Near the terminal segment of a seminiferous tubule, the spermatogenic cells decrease in number and the Sertoli cells become more numerous. A **transitional zone**, lined by Sertoli cells, joins a seminiferous tubule to a **straight tubule**. The latter may be lined by simple columnar, cuboidal, or squamous cells and is continuous with a network of anastomosing channels that form the **rete testis**. The rete testis possesses a simple squamous or cuboidal epithelium that may be bistratified cuboidal in the bull. It is surrounded by the loose connective tissue of the **mediastinum testis**.

Efferent ductules, lined by a simple columnar or a pseudostratified epithelium with some ciliated cells, lead from the rete testis and pass through the tunica albuginea to join the **duct of the epididymis** in the head of the **epididymis**. In the stallion the tubules of the rete testis penetrate the tunica albuginea and form an **extratesticular rete testis,** which is then joined to the duct of the epididymis by efferent ductules. The coiled duct of the epididymis varies in structure from the head to the tail region of the epididymis. Its pseudostratified columnar epithelium, with stereocilia, is thickest in the head region and is encircled by some smooth muscle. In the body (mid) region there is less smooth muscle, and the epithelium is thinner. In the tail region of the epididymis the pseudostratified epithelium is thinnest, and the surrounding smooth muscle is most abundant. In the stallion the lining of the duct in the tail region of the epididymis forms short, villuslike projections.

The **vas deferens** (ductus deferens) leads from the duct of the epididymis and joins with the urethra. The vas deferens is lined by a pseudostratified columnar epithelium (some cells with stereocilia) that may become simple columnar distally. The smooth muscle of its thick muscularis presents a variety of arrangements. It may form an inner circular and an outer longitudinal layer, and each of these layers may contain interwoven fibers of smooth muscle. In contrast, the entire muscularis may be interwoven with no distinct layers of smooth muscle. We have not observed any particular arrangement to be consistent within a species.

The **male accessory glands** include the glands of the ampulla, seminal vesicles, the bulbourethral glands, and the prostate gland. They are composed of branched tubular or tubuloacinar secretory units that often have vesicular dilations. The secretory epithelium of these glands is classified as pseudostratified because, although consisting primarily of columnar cells (or sometimes cuboidal cells such as in the prostate), occasional basal cells are present.

Near its junction with the urethra, the vas deferens forms a dilated **ampulla** whose lamina propria and submucosa are filled with glandular secretory units. The ampulla is absent in the tomcat, and the ampullary glands are not well developed in the boar.

The **prostate gland** is a seromucous gland except in the dog, where it is entirely serous. In the boar and ruminants, the prostate gland consists mostly of a **disseminate portion** (pars disseminata) in the form of a glandular layer in the submucosa of the pelvic urethra. In the stallion and carnivores the disseminate portion is represented only by scattered glands. The **body of the prostate gland** is well developed in the stallion and carnivore and is absent in the ram and billy goat (buck). It is an encapsulated, lobulated gland that partially or completely surrounds a part of the pelvic urethra.

The **seminal vesicles** (vesicular glands) are absent in carnivores. In the stallion they are true vesicular outpocketings in the form of bladderlike sacs with wide central lumens into which the glands open. In the boar and ruminants they are compact glands with a lobulated surface.

The mucous-secreting **bulbourethral** (Cowper's) **glands** are present in all domestic mammals except the dog. The columnar cells of the pseudostratified epithelium are tall and pale and possess basally displaced nuclei.

The male **urethra,** which carries both urine and semen, can be divided into a pelvic and a penile portion. The **pelvic urethra** is lined by a transitional epithelium, which may become stratified columnar or cuboidal distally. Along the entire length of the urethra, the connective tissue below the mucosa contains erectile tissue with thin-walled **cavernous spaces** (veins). In the pelvic urethra this erectile tissue forms the **stratum cavernosum** (vascular stratum). Peripheral to this stratum are the glands of the disseminate portion of the prostate gland. The muscularis of the urethra near the bladder consists of an inner and outer longitudinal layer and a middle circular layer of smooth muscle. In the vicinity of the prostate gland, most of the smooth muscle is replaced by skeletal urethral muscle. However, some longitudinal smooth muscle remains. The muscularis of the pelvic urethra is surrounded by an adventitia.

The **penile urethra,** which courses through the ventral region of the penis, is lined by a mixture of transitional, stratified cuboidal, stratified columnar, or simple columnar epithelium. The larger, more abundant cavernous spaces of the penile urethra form the **corpus spongiosum** (corpus cavernosum urethra), which is surrounded by a tunica albuginea. Except for an occasional cell, the wall of the penile urethra lacks a muscularis of smooth muscle.

In the stallion and ruminants the terminal portion of the urethra extends beyond the penis, forming a **urethral process**. It is covered by a cutaneous membrane and lined by transitional or stratified squamous epithelium. In the stallion the urethral process contains well-developed erectile tissue. In the ram and billy goat the urethral process contains small cavernous spaces and two cords of fibrocartilage that parallel the urethra.

The **penis** can be divided into the body and glans penis. Both regions contain the penile urethra with its erectile tissue, the corpus spongiosum. The **body of the penis** (corpus penis) is characterized by two additional masses of erectile tissue called the **corpora cavernosa**. Each corpus cavernosum is enclosed by the dense connective tissue and elastic fibers of the tunica albuginea. The tunic is especially thick in the boar and ruminants and contains smooth muscle in the stallion. It extends inward to form a network of trabeculae between which lies the spongy erectile tissue. The latter contains cavernous spaces, lined by endothelium and surrounded by various proportions of smooth muscle and fibroelastic connective tissue. In the vascular penis of the stallion the smooth muscle is predominant. In the fibroelastic penis of the boar and ruminants the cavernous spaces are surrounded mainly by connective tissue that is rich in elastic fibers and contains little or no smooth muscle. In the intermediate type of penis of the carnivore, both smooth muscle and connective tissue fill the spaces between the cavernous vessels. The corpus cavernosum of all domestic mammals contains scattered adipose tissue in the connective tissue between the cavernous vessels. This is abundant in the tomcat, especially toward the tip of the corpus cavernosum, where adipose tissue nearly replaces the erectile tissue.

The cavernous spaces receive their blood supply from groups of **helicine arteries**. The walls of these tortuous vessels have cushionlike thickenings, formed from longitudinal bundles of smooth muscle, epithelioid cells, and abundant elastic tissue.

The expanded, distal portion of the penis, called the **glans penis,** is best developed in the stallion and dog. It contains erectile tissue, which is continuous with that of the corpus spongiosum. In carnivores the glans contains an **os penis**. This bone is small in the tomcat. It is well developed in the dog and possesses a fibrocartilaginous tip. The surface (visceral prepuce) of the glans penis of the tomcat bears small, keratinized epidermal spines. Small epidermal projections also occur in the stallion and billy goat.

The **prepuce** is a tubelike reflection of skin that covers the distal, free portion of the penis. It is composed of an external, parietal, and visceral layer. The external layer is typical skin and is continuous with the abdominal skin. The external layer turns inward at the preputial opening to form the parietal prepuce (internal layer). This, in turn, reflects at the fornix and continues onto the end of the penis as the visceral prepuce. The stallion has an additional outer fold called the sheath. Hair, sweat glands, and sebaceous glands occur over a variable distance from the external layer to the parietal prepuce. Glands may occur occasionally in the visceral prepuce of the stallion.

CHICKEN

The **testes** are situated in the abdominal cavity of the rooster. They are surrounded by a thin connective-tissue capsule, the **tunica albuginea,** which is covered by a **peritoneum.** There are no well-developed septa to divide the testes into lobules.

The epithelial cells of the convoluted **seminiferous tubules** are like those of mammals: Sertoli cells, spermatogonia, primary spermatocytes, secondary spermatocytes, spermatids, and spermatozoa. Unlike those in mammals, various cell associations do not occur in segments along the length of the seminiferous tubules. Instead, the seminiferous epithelium is arranged into narrow columns of cells that undergo spermatogenesis independently. There is very little connective tissue between adjacent seminiferous tubules, and **interstitial cells** are sparse. They occur singly or in small clusters, primarily in the larger interstitial spaces. They are flattened to polyhedral cells with a relatively large, round nucleus and cytoplasm that is often vacuolated.

The seminiferous tubules are continuous with **straight tubules,** which are lined by Sertoli cells. Straight tubules lead into the anastomosing channels of the **rete testis,** which is lined by a simple cuboidal to squamous epithelium. The rete testis lies outside the tunica albuginea below the epididymis.

Three types of tubules occur within the **epididymis:** efferent ductules, connecting ducts, and the duct of the epididymis. The numerous, convoluted **efferent ductules** join the rete testis to the connecting ducts. They are lined by a simple epithelium of intermittent groups of tall and low, columnar cells, as well as patches of cells that appear to be pseudostratified. The epithelial cells are arranged into folds, and many of the cells bear tufts of cilia. The **connecting ducts** (excretory canals) are smaller in diameter than the other tubules of the epididymis and are lined by a pseudostratified columnar epithelium. The epithelial cells are rarely ciliated and are not arranged into numerous folds as are the cells that line the efferent ductules. Thus, the luminal surface of the connecting ducts has a smooth appearance. The single, convoluted **duct of the epididymis** is similar in structure to the connecting ducts, except that it is much larger in diameter. All of the tubules of the epididymis are surrounded and bound by connective tissue.

At the terminal portion of the epididymis, the duct of the epididymis joins the **vas deferens.** The latter is a convoluted duct with a pseudostratified columnar epithelium, underlying smooth muscle, and a more peripheral layer of dense connective tissue. Each vas deferens merges with a small, conical **ejaculatory duct,** whose submucosa contains erectile tissue. The ejaculatory duct protrudes and opens into the urodeum of the **cloaca,** marking the termination of the duct system of the male.

Figure 17.1   ×18

Figure 17.2   ×90

KEY	
1. Gonocyte	4. Sex cord
2. Interstitial cells	5. Straight tubule
3. Rete testis	6. Supporting cells

Figure 17.1. Testis, x.s., Baby Boar. Developing sex cords in the testis of a two-day-old boar.

Figure 17.2. Testis, x.s., Baby Boar. Detail of developing sex cords and interstitial cells. Two types of cells can be distinguished in the sex cord. Supporting cells (small with dark nuclei) are positioned along the edges of the cords. They will develop into Sertoli cells. Gonocytes, precursors of spermatogonia, are located in the interior of the cords. They have large, pale nuclei.

Figure 17.3

×25

Figure 17.4

×25

KEY	
1. Interstitial cells	8. Spermatid, late
2. Lumen	9. Spermatogonia
3. Myoid cell, nucleus	10. Tunica albuginea
4. Primary spermatocyte	11. Tunica albuginea, smooth muscle
5. Seminiferous tubule	12. Tunica albuginea, vascular layer
6. Sertoli cell, nucleus	13. Tunica vaginalis
7. Spermatid, early	

Figure 17.3. Testis, Stallion (Mallory's). The tunica albuginea of the stallion is characterized by the presence of smooth muscle.

Figure 17.4. Testis, Boar (Mallory's). The tunica albuginea consists of dense irregular connective tissue. It lacks smooth muscle in domestic mammals, except the stallion.

Figure 17.5. Seminiferous Tubules, Testis, Dog. A portion of each of three adjacent seminiferous tubules is shown.

Figure 17.5

×360

Figure 17.6 ×180

Figure 17.9 ×12.5

KEY		
1. Efferent ductule	9.	Sertoli cells
2. Interstitial cell	10.	Spermatid, early
3. Mediastinum testis	11.	Spermatid, late
4. Myoid cell, nucleus	12.	Spermatogonium
5. Primary spermatocyte	13.	Straight tubule
6. Rete testis, channel	14.	Transitional zone
7. Seminiferous tubules	15.	Tunica albuginea
8. Sertoli cell, nucleus		

Figure 17.6. Seminiferous Tubules, Testis, Stallion. Portions of four seminiferous tubules are visible. Note the numerous interstitial cells (abundant in the boar and stallion) and the section through a straight tubule.

Figure 17.7. Interstitial Tissue, Testis, Ram. Interstitial tissue and portions of three seminiferous tubules are shown. Interstitial cells are relatively sparse in carnivores and ruminants.

Figure 17.8. Transitional Zone and Straight Tubule, Testis, Stallion. A transitional zone joins a seminiferous tubule to a straight tubule. Sertoli cells line this zone and protrude into the lumen of the straight tubule.

Figure 17.9. Rete Testis, Stallion. Anastomosing channels of the rete testis lie within the loose connective tissue of the mediastinum testis. In the stallion the rete testis extends through the tunica albuginea and becomes extratesticular, as in this micrograph. Junctions of rete channels and efferent ductules can be seen. See Figure 17.10 for a magnified view of a junction.

Figure 17.7 ×250

Figure 17.8 ×125

Figure 17.10 ×250

Figure 17.11 ×25

Figure 17.12 ×250

Figure 17.13 ×25

Figure 17.14 ×62.5

KEY	
1. Columnar epithelium	8. Pseudostratified epithelium, efferent ductule
2. Cuboidal epithelium, rete testis	9. Smooth muscle
3. Duct of the epididymis	10. Spermatozoa
4. Efferent ductule	11. Tunica albuginea, smooth muscle
5. Loose connective tissue	12. Tunica vaginalis, mesothelium
6. Lymphocyte, migrating	
7. Pseudostratified epithelium	

Figure 17.10. Junction of Rete Testis and Efferent Ductule, Stallion. The rete testis is lined by cuboidal cells, whereas the efferent ductule is lined by a ciliated, pseudostratified columnar epithelium.

Figure 17.11. Efferent Ductules, Stallion. Various cuts through the tortuous efferent ductules are surrounded by loose connective tissue.

Figure 17.12. Efferent Ductules, Stallion. Efferent ductules are lined by a ciliated, pseudostratified columnar epithelium. However, the epithelium may be simple columnar in some places.

Figure 17.13. Head of Epididymis, Stallion (Masson's). The epididymis is surrounded by a tunica albuginea of dense irregular connective tissue, which contains smooth muscle in the stallion. Portions of the coiled duct of the epididymis are shown.

Figure 17.14. Head of Epididymis, Stallion. In this region the pseudostratified columnar epithelium of the duct of the epididymis is thickest. Smooth muscle is scarce. Compare with Figures 17.15 and 17.16.

Figure 17.15   ×62.5

Figure 17.19   ×62.5

Figure 17.16   ×62.5

KEY		
1. Basal cell	6.	Serosa
2. Lamina propria	7.	Smooth muscle
3. Loose connective tissue	8.	Spermatozoa
4. Muscularis	9.	Stereocilia
5. Pseudostratified epithelium	10.	Villus-like projection

Figure 17.15. Body of Epididymis, Stallion. The duct of the epididymis in this region is surrounded by more smooth muscle than in the head of the epididymis, and the pseudostratified columnar epithelium is not as thick as in the head of the epididymis (see Fig. 17.14).

Figure 17.16. Tail of Epididymis, Stallion. A low, pseudostratified columnar epithelium and abundant circular smooth muscle characterize the duct of the epididymis in this region. In the stallion the caudal segment of the duct of the epididymis has villuslike projections.

Figure 17.17. Tail of Epididymis, Stallion. Detail of the duct of the epididymis lined by low, pseudostratified columnar epithelium and surrounded by abundant, circular smooth muscle.

Figure 17.18. Vas Deferens, x.s., Dog. The bulk of the wall consists of smooth muscle, which forms an inner circular and an outer predominantly longitudinal layer with some randomly arranged cells.

Figure 17.19. Vas Deferens, x.s., Stallion (Masson's). This section of the vas deferens, taken from near the epididymis, has long mucosal folds. The inner layer of the muscularis contains interwoven bundles of smooth muscle. Although out of the field of view in this micrograph, the smooth muscle of the outer layer of the muscularis is mostly arranged longitudinally.

Figure 17.17   ×250

Figure 17.18   ×25

Figure 17.20   ×62.5

Figure 17.21   ×12.5

Figure 17.22   ×62.5

Figure 17.23   ×125

Figure 17.24   ×25

KEY	
1. Adventitia	7. Muscularis
2. Ampulla, lumen	8. Pseudostratified epithelium
3. Basal cell, nucleus	9. Secretion
4. Gland	10. Serosa
5. Interlobular septum	11. Spermatozoa
6. Lamina propria	

Figure 17.20. Vas Deferens, x.s., Boar (Masson's). The muscularis consists of an admixture of longitudinally and randomly arranged smooth muscle. The epithelium is pseudostratified columnar with stereocilia present intermittently.

Figure 17.21. Ampulla, x.s., Ram. The terminal segment of the vas deferens, the ampulla, contains branched tubuloalveolar glands in the dog, stallion, and ruminants. The glands are poorly developed in the boar. The ampulla is absent in the tomcat.

Figure 17.22. Ampulla, Ram. Detail of the mucosa. Spermatozoa are stored in the glands close to their openings into the lumen of the ampulla.

Figure 17.23. Ampulla, Ram. The secretory alveoli are lined by a pseudostratified epithelium composed of cuboidal to columnar cells and occasional basal cells.

Figure 17.24. Seminal Vesicle, Castrated Billy Goat. In the castrated male the glandular tissue of the accessory glands is greatly reduced. Compare with Figure 17.25.

MALE REPRODUCTIVE SYSTEM   **211**

Figure 17.25 ×25

Figure 17.29 ×12.5

Figure 17.26 ×250

Figure 17.25. Seminal Vesicle, Ram. Lobules of tubuloalveolar glands are divided by interlobular septa, which contain an abundance of smooth muscle in ruminants. In the stallion and boar the septa consist predominantly of connective tissue with some smooth muscle. Seminal vesicles are absent in carnivores.

Figure 17.26. Seminal Vesicle, Ram. The pseudostratified glandular epithelium is characterized by sparse basal cells. Note the muscular septum.

Figure 17.27. Body of the Prostate, Dog. The body of the prostate, which is well developed in carnivores and the stallion, is surrounded by a capsule of dense connective tissue and smooth muscle. Trabeculae from the capsule divide the gland into lobules.

Figure 17.28. Body of the Prostate, Dog. In the dog, this is a serous gland. Compare with Figure 17.31.

Figure 17.29. Disseminate Portion of the Prostate, x.s., Ram (Masson's). This portion of the prostate is well developed in the boar and ruminants. The glands are located within the submucosa of the pelvic urethra. The stratum cavernosum of the pelvic urethra contains cavernous spaces that are smaller and less numerous than those of the corpus spongiosum of the penile urethra.

Figure 17.27 ×12.5

Figure 17.28 ×62.5

Figure 17.30

×125

Figure 17.33

×12.5

Figure 17.31

×125

Figure 17.34

×62.5

Figure 17.32

×36

KEY	
1. Cavernous space	7. Secretory cells
2. Corpus spongiosum	8. Serous cells
3. Duct	9. Smooth muscle
4. Lamina propria	10. Spongy bone
5. Mucous cells	11. Transitional epithelium
6. Os penis	12. Urethra, lumen

Figure 17.30. Disseminate Portion of the Prostate, x.s., Ram (Masson's). The transitional epithelium of both the pelvic urethra and a duct of the prostate gland is shown.

Figure 17.31. Disseminate Portion of the Prostate, x.s., Ram (Masson's). The prostate is a mixed gland except in the dog, where there are no mucous secretory units.

Figure 17.32. Bulbourethral Gland, Boar. This gland is a compound tubular gland in the boar, tomcat, and billy goat. It is a tubuloalveolar gland in the stallion, bull, and ram. It is absent in the dog. The pale-staining secretory cells are columnar or pyramidal and have basally displaced nuclei.

Figure 17.33. Penis, x.s., Puppy. Section is through the developing os penis, which is present in carnivores.

Figure 17.34. Penis, x.s., Puppy. Detail of the urethra and portion of the os penis.

Figure 17.35 ×12.5

Figure 17.39 ×125

Figure 17.36 ×62.5

KEY	
1. Cavernous space	8. Lamina propria
2. Connective tissue	9. Os penis
3. Corpus cavernosum	10. Smooth muscle
4. Corpus spongiosum	11. Stratified columnar epithelium
5. Dermis	12. Tunica albuginea
6. Endothelium	13. Urethra, lumen
7. Epidermal spine	

Figure 17.35. Penis, l.s., Tomcat. In the tomcat the distal portion of the corpus cavernosum consists largely of nonerectile, adipose tissue. A small os penis is present in the glans, and small spines are present on the surface of the glans of the tomcat. (Photomicrograph of a histologic section borrowed from the College of Veterinary Medicine, Iowa State University.)

Figure 17.36. Glans Penis, l.s., Tomcat. Detail of a keratinized epidermal spine. (Photomicrograph of a histologic section borrowed from the College of Veterinary Medicine, Iowa State University.)

Figure 17.37. Penile Urethra, x.s., Stallion. Portion of the penile urethra with abundant cavernous spaces of the corpus spongiosum.

Figure 17.38. Corpus Spongiosum, Body of Penis, Stallion. The cavernous spaces of the stallion and carnivore are surrounded by connective tissue rich in elastic fibers and by many bundles of smooth muscle.

Figure 17.39. Penile Urethra, x.s., Stallion. The epithelial lining of the urethra in this section is stratified columnar. The epithelium, however, is variable in the penile urethra and in places may also be simple columnar, transitional, or stratified cuboidal.

Figure 17.37 ×12.5

Figure 17.38 ×62.5

Figure 17.40 ×12.5

Figure 17.44 ×25

Figure 17.41 ×12.5

KEY	
1. Adipose tissue	6. Elastic fibers
2. Cavernous space	7. Retractor penis muscle
3. Connective tissue	8. Smooth muscle
4. Connective tissue trabecula	9. Tunica albuginea
5. Corpus cavernosum	10. Urethra, lumen

Figure 17.40. Body of Penis, Stallion. Large masses of smooth muscle surround the cavernous spaces of the corpus cavernosum of the stallion.

Figure 17.41. Body of Penis, x.s., Boar. A portion of the sigmoid flexure, including the retractor penis muscle.

Figure 17.42. Body of Penis, x.s., Boar (Orcein). The connective tissue surrounding the cavernous spaces of the corpus cavernosum is rich in elastic fibers in the boar and ruminants.

Figure 17.43. Body of Penis, Boar. In the boar and ruminant the cavernous spaces of the corpus cavernosum are invested largely by connective tissue and only a smattering of smooth muscle.

Figure 17.44. Penile Urethra, x.s., Ram. The distribution of the cavernous spaces of the corpus spongiosum of the penile urethra is especially well represented in this section.

Figure 17.42 ×25

Figure 17.43 ×62.5

MALE REPRODUCTIVE SYSTEM **215**

Figure 17.45 ×62.5

Figure 17.46 ×25

Figure 17.47 ×62.5

Figure 17.48 ×62.5

Figure 17.49 ×12.5

KEY	
1. Cavernous space	8. Smooth muscle
2. Elastic fibers	9. Stratified squamous epithelium
3. Epidermis	10. Trabecula
4. Fibrocartilaginous cord	11. Transitional epithelium
5. Helicine artery	12. Tunica albuginea
6. Lamina propria	13. Urethra, lumen
7. Smegma	

Figure 17.45. Body of Penis, x.s., Ram (Orcein). The cavernous spaces of the corpus spongiosum are surrounded by connective tissue rich in elastic fibers in boars and ruminants.

Figure 17.46. Helicine Artery, Body of Penis, Ram (Orcein). The corpus cavernosum contains helicine arteries, which are tortuous vessels with an abundance of elastic fibers throughout their walls.

Figure 17.47. Helicine Artery, Body of Penis, Ram (Masson's). Junction of a helicine artery with a cavernous space in the corpus cavernosum.

Figure 17.48. Urethral Process, x.s., Ram. The urethral process is a tortuous, wormlike extension of the urethra in the ram and billy goat. One of the two fibrocartilaginous cords that parallel the urethra is shown.

Figure 17.49. Urethral Pouch, Stallion. The urethral pouch, found only in the stallion, is filled with smegma, which is composed of desquamated epithelial cells and the secretion of the preputial glands.

Figure 17.50 ×25

Figure 17.51 ×25

Figure 17.52 ×18

Figure 17.53 ×250

KEY	
1. Connecting duct	10. Rete testis
2. Dermal papilla	11. Sebaceous gland
3. Efferent ductule	12. Seminiferous tubule
4. Hair follicle	13. Sertoli cell, nucleus
5. Interstitial cell	14. Spermatid, early
6. Lymphatic nodule	15. Spermatid, late
7. Parietal prepuce	16. Spermatogonium
8. Preputial gland	17. Stratified squamous epithelium
9. Primary spermatocyte	18. Visceral prepuce

Figure 17.50. Parietal Prepuce, Stallion. The dermis contains sebaceous glands and tubular preputial (sweat) glands.

Figure 17.51. Prepuce, Boar. The parietal and visceral prepuce are shown.

Figure 17.52. Testis and Epididymis, x.s., Rooster. Seminiferous tubules, the rete testis, and portions (efferent ductules and connecting ducts) of the epididymis.

Figure 17.53. Interstitial Tissue, Testis, Rooster. Interstitial (Leydig) cells are found principally in the larger intertubular spaces. These cells are either polyhedral or elongated and may contain vacuoles.

Figure 17.54

×360

Figure 17.57

×250

Figure 17.54. Seminiferous Tubules, Testis, Rooster. Detail of portions of adjacent seminiferous tubules. Note that the seminiferous epithelial cells are organized into narrow columns.

Figure 17.55. Testis, Rooster. A straight tubule, lined by Sertoli cells, connects a seminiferous tubule with the rete testis.

Figure 17.56. Straight Tubule, Testis, Rooster. Sertoli cells form the epithelium of straight tubules.

Figure 17.57. Junction of Rete Testis and Efferent Ductule, Rooster. The epithelial cells lining efferent ductules vary in shape and many possess cilia. The rete testis is lined by squamous epithelial cells.

Figure 17.55

×62.5

Figure 17.56

×250

Figure 17.58   ×250

Figure 17.59   ×250

Figure 17.60   ×62.5

Figure 17.61   ×125

KEY	
1. Cilia	5. Pseudostratified epithelium
2. Connecting duct	6. Smooth muscle
3. Duct of the epididymis	7. Spermatozoa
4. Efferent ductule	

Figure 17.58. Efferent Ductule, x.s., Rooster. Detail of an efferent ductule. The epithelial cells vary in shape, and many bear cilia. The epithelium is folded and is surrounded by loose connective tissue. Occasionally, smooth muscle may be present.

Figure 17.59. Connecting Duct and Efferent Ductule, Rooster. Connecting ducts present a smooth inner surface and are lined by a pseudostratified columnar epithelium with occasional basal cells. The epithelial cells are generally without cilia. In contrast, the efferent ductule has a folded lining, and its epithelial cells are mostly ciliated.

Figure 17.60. Duct of the Epididymis, Rooster. The duct of the epididymis has a larger diameter than a connecting duct, but otherwise is comparable in structure with the latter.

Figure 17.61. Vas Deferens, Distal, Rooster. The lining epithelium is similar to that of the epididymis. A layer of smooth muscle separates the epithelium from the surrounding connective tissue.

18

FEMALE REPRODUCTIVE SYSTEM

MAMMALS

The ovaries, oviducts, uterus, vagina, and vulva are the major components of the mammalian female reproductive system. A simple squamous or cuboidal epithelium, **germinal epithelium,** often missing from histologic preparations, covers the **cortex** of the **ovary.** Beneath the epithelium is a layer of dense connective tissue, the **tunica albuginea.** A **cortical stroma,** containing ovarian **follicles** in various stages of development, lies internal to the tunica albuginea. In bitches and queens, but ordinarily not in other domestic mammals, cords of epithelioid cells called **interstitial glands** occur throughout the stroma. The epithelioid cells are derived from the theca interna of atretic, antral follicles or from the granulosa cells of atretic, preantral follicles.

A **medulla** consisting of richly vascularized loose connective tissue lies internal to the ovarian cortex. In the mare the medullary tissue is located external to the cortex. Channels, lined by a cuboidal epithelium and called the **rete ovarii,** are conspicuous components of the medulla in carnivores and ruminants. **Hilus cells** (groups of epithelioid cells) may be found close to the rete ovarii in the region of the hilus in some mammals.

Primordial follicles are the least developed and most numerous follicles of the ovary. They lie just below the tunica albuginea. Each consists of a **primary oocyte** surrounded by a layer of simple squamous **follicle cells.** In response to periodic hormonal stimulation, growth is initiated in some of the primordial follicles. The earliest growing follicle, the **primary follicle,** consists of an enlarging oocyte surrounded by a layer of cuboidal cells. Proliferation of the follicle cells results in the formation of a **multilaminar** (late primary) **follicle.** Fluid-filled spaces appearing between the follicle cells gradually coalesce, forming an antrum. Concomitantly, an acidophilic, translucent membrane, the **zona pellucida,** appears around the oocyte. Further growth results in the formation of a **secondary follicle** with a C-shaped **antrum.** Its follicle cells are now called the **membrana granulosa.** A sheath of stromal cells, the **theca folliculi,** forms around the follicle. The theca differentiates into a cellular, vascular inner layer, the **theca interna,** and an outer layer of connective tissue, the **theca externa.** The boundary between the stroma and the theca externa and

221

that between the theca externa and theca interna is often indistinct. Continued growth results in the formation of a large **tertiary** (Graafian) **follicle** whose oocyte is surrounded by a multilayer of membrana granulosa cells, the **cumulus oophorus.** The columnar cells of the innermost portion of the latter constitute the **corona radiata,** which is separated from the oocyte by the zona pellucida.

Ordinarily, each mature tertiary follicle contains a single oocyte. The follicles of certain animals (carnivores, sows, and ewes) may, however, contain as many as six oocytes.

Mature follicles vary widely in size. They are about 2 mm in diameter in the bitch and queen, 15 mm in the cow, and as large as 70 mm in the mare. Maximum size is reached just prior to ovulation. Following ovulation, granulosa cells and cells of the theca interna of most species multiply, hypertrophy, and differentiate into granulosa lutein cells and smaller, more peripheral theca lutein cells, respectively, of the **corpus luteum.** A yellow pigment (lutein) is formed by the luteal cells of the cow, mare, and carnivores, but is lacking in ewes, nanny goats (does), and sows. Luteal cells produce progesterone. Regression of the corpus luteum occurs during late diestrus, leaving scar tissue, the **corpus albicans.**

Although many primordial follicles begin the process of growth and differentiation, few become mature. The majority undergo a degenerative regression, called **atresia.** The oocyte and membrane granulosa degenerate first. Cells of the theca interna hypertrophy, and the zona pellucida becomes swollen. Eventually, the entire follicle is resorbed.

The **oviduct** is a muscular tube consisting of an **isthmus,** which arises from the uterus; a middle segment, the **ampulla;** and a funnel-shaped **infundibulum,** which lies next to the ovary. From the outside inward, the wall of the oviduct is comprised of a serosa, muscularis, lamina propria, and epithelium. The muscularis, which is thickest in the isthmus, is formed mainly from circular smooth muscle with a modicum of longitudinally arranged smooth muscle external to it. Many of the epithelial cells lining the cavity of the oviduct are ciliated. In part, the epithelium of ruminants and sows is pseudostratified. The mucosa is thrown into longitudinal folds, with less folding occurring in the isthmus than in the ampulla.

The wall of the bicornuate **uterus** of domestic mammals has three layers: the outer **perimetrium** (serosa), middle **myometrium,** and inner **endometrium** (mucosa). The myometrium is divisible into a thick, inner circular layer and a thin, outer longitudinal layer. A richly vascularized and well-innervated **stratum vasculare** usually separates the muscle layers. The stratum vasculare, however, is indistinct in the sow and may be located in the outer half of the circular layer in the cow.

The epithelium of the endometrium is simple cuboidal or columnar in the bitch, queen, and mare, but may be stratified or pseudostratified in ruminants and sows. Simple, branched **uterine** (endometrial) **glands** extend into the lamina propria. These may be considerably coiled in the mare, sow, and ruminants. Nonglandular regions of the endometrium, called **caruncles,** occur in ruminants.

The mucosa of the uterine **cervix** is elevated into longitudinal folds that may become subdivided into secondary and tertiary folds. The epithelial lining is simple columnar with goblet cells. In the bitch, however, it is stratified squamous. Glandular tissue fades in the cervix, extending to the cervical os only in carnivores. An inner circular and an outer longitudinal layer of smooth muscle form the muscularis.

The **estrous cycle** consists of a succession of stages. The first stage, **proestrus,** is characterized by endometrial growth. It is followed by **estrus,** or period when the female is receptive to the male. In most species, ovulation occurs during estrus. The development of the corpus luteum occurs during the next stage, **metestrus. Diestrus** follows metestrus and coincides with the presence of a fully functional corpus luteum. During this time the development and secretory activity of the endometrial glands peak. **Anestrus,** a period of sexual inactivity, follows diestrus.

The **placenta** is derived from the endometrium and the chorioallantoic membrane (CAM). The degree of intimacy between these two components varies and is a basis for classifying placentas. A placenta is **indeciduate** when these two membranes are in contact but are not intimately fused. The placenta is **deciduate** when the membranes have become fused. Little or no endometrium is lost during the birth process in animals having an indeciduate placenta (mare, ruminants, and sow). Conversely, considerable mucosa is lost at parturition in animals with deciduate placentas (carnivores).

The extent to which the CAM contributes to the placenta is variable. If most of the CAM contributes, as in the mare and sow, the placenta is **diffuse;** if numerous but isolated areas contribute, as in ruminants, the placenta is **cotyledonary;** when a beltlike portion of the CAM contributes, as in carnivores, the placenta is **zonary.**

The surfaces of the chorioallantoic membrane and the endometrium may contact one another in three different ways. These types of contact are designated as **folded, villous,** and **labyrinthine.** In the sow both surfaces are folded and are closely applied to each other. In the mare and ruminants chorioallantoic villi insert into pockets (crypts) in the endometrium. In carnivores the apposed surfaces form a complex, interlinked, fused labyrinth.

Classification of the placenta can also be based on the number of tissue layers separating the fetal and maternal blood. In the mare and sow six layers intervene: the endothelium, connective tissue, and epithelium of the CAM; and the epithelium, connective tissue, and endothelium of the endometrium. This configuration characterizes the **epitheliochorial placenta.** In ewes and nanny goats (does) the epithelium of the **caruncles** (endometrial elevations where functional contact with the CAM is made) is lost, thereby reducing the number of tissue layers to five (**syndesmochorial placenta**). In the cow the epithelium of the caruncle remains intact (epitheliochorial), but portions of the intercaruncular epithelium degenerate. In carnivores both the endometrial epithelium and the endometrial connective tissue are lost, bringing the epithelium of the CAM and the endothelium of the endometrium into contact. Only four tissue layers separate the fetal and maternal blood in this type, the **endotheliochorial placenta.**

A mucosa, muscularis, and adventitia or serosa (cranial region only) form the wall of the **vagina.** The mucosa is lined, throughout, by a stratified squamous epithelium in all species except the cow. In the anterior portion of the vagina of the cow, the epithelium is stratified columnar with goblet cells. In carnivores, the epithelial cells become keratinized during estrus. A lamina propria and submucosa are present. Usually, the inner layer of the muscularis is thick and consists of circularly arranged smooth muscle, while the outer layer is thin and consists of longitudinally organized smooth muscle. In some animals (bitch, queen, and sow) a thin layer of longitudinal muscle occurs internal to the circular layer. An adventitia or serosa is present.

Vaginal cytology provides a way of determining stages of the estrous cycle of the bitch or queen and therefore can be helpful to the practitioner who is trying to determine the best time to breed an animal. In the bitch, for example, **proestrus, estrus, diestrus,** and **anestrus** are stages of the estrous cycle. The formation of the corpus luteum occurs during late estrus in the bitch. Therefore, there is no **metestrus.** Proestrus lasts an average of 9 days and is characterized by a watery, bloody discharge and swollen vulva. Estrus is evidenced when a bitch is willing to stand for mating, and ordinarily lasts about 9 days. A clear or bloody discharge is present. Diestrus lasts for about 2 months and begins on the day when the bitch no longer tolerates a male's advances. Anestrus follows diestrus and may last from two to ten months.

Various types of epithelial cells are found in vaginal smears taken during the estrous cycle. **Parabasal cells** are the smallest. They are round cells with round nuclei, and have the highest nucleocytoplasmic ratio of any of the sloughed cells. **Intermediate cells** are larger than parabasal cells. Their nuclei are similar in size and shape to those of the latter. The corners of intermediate cells are rounded. **Superficial intermediate cells** (transitional cells) are bigger than intermediate cells and have angular edges. Their nuclei resemble those of parabasal and intermediate cells. **Superficial cells** are similar in size to superficial intermediate cells. Their edges are angular and may be folded. Their nuclei are pyknotic, faded, or lacking.

Smears taken during proestrus (early to mid) may contain erythrocytes and neutrophils as well as parabasal, intermediate, superficial intermediate, and superficial cells. During late proestrus, superficial intermediate and superficial cells are the most numerous, and neutrophils decline.

The vast majority (90% or more) of cells found in smears taken during estrus are superficial cells. During late proestrus, similar smears may be obtained. Ordinarily, during estrus, neutrophils are not observed. Erythrocytes show a reduction in number, but in many bitches they can be found throughout estrus and into early diestrus. Bacteria may be found in estrous smears.

During diestrus, superficial cells decrease by a minimum of twenty percent. Parabasal and intermediate cells, which may have been absent or very sparse, increase to more than 10% and frequently rise to more than 50%. Although neutrophils reappear during diestrus, smears from some bitches contain few or none. Because erythrocytes may be present in smears from early diestrus, it is not possible to distinguish proestrus from diestrus without taking more than one smear.

During anestrus, parabasal and intermediate cells predominate in smears. Bacteria may be found, but will be less abundant than in proestrus or estrus. Neutrophils may occur, but are ordinarily less abundant than in early diestrus.

In domestic mammals, the **vulva** includes the **vestibule, labia,** and **clitoris.** The mucosal epithelium is stratified squamous. The major vestibular glands are bilateral, mucus-secreting, tubuloacinar glands in the submucosa, found in ruminants and the queen. Minor vestibular glands occur in the mucosa of most domestic animals. They are small, branched, tubular, mucous glands distributed through the vestibular mucosa.

The integument of the labia (lips of the vulva) has a structure like that of the external skin. It is well endowed with both sebaceous and tubular apocrine glands.

The clitoris consists of **erectile tissue** (corpus cavernosum clitoridis), a **glans,** and a **prepuce.** The amount of erectile tissue varies. The prepuce has parietal and visceral components as in males.

CHICKEN

The left **ovary** and oviduct represent the reproductive organs of the hen. The ovary consists of an outer **cortex** that envelops a vascular **medulla.** Ovarian follicles of various sizes occur within the cortex. A layer (germinal epithelium) of cuboidal or flattened cells covers the cortex. The **tunica albuginea,** composed of dense connective tissue, lies below the epithelium. A **stroma** of loose connective tissue occurs below the tunica albuginea.

Developing follicles occur throughout the stroma of the cortex. Large follicles are suspended from the surface of the ovary by stalks of cortical tissue. Each follicle consists of a growing, yolk-laden oocyte with a rounded nucleus (**germinal vesicle**). The oocyte is surrounded by several layers. These are, from the outside inward, the **theca externa, theca interna, membrana granulosa,** and **perivitelline membrane.** The latter abuts the surface membrane of the oocyte.

The theca externa is formed from a compact connective tissue that contains groups of pale **interstitial** (luteal) **cells.** The latter may also be found, in groups, in the cortical stroma and medulla. The theca interna is only about one quarter as thick as the externa. It is formed from a compact layer of spindle-shaped cells. The membrana granulosa consists of a single layer of cuboidal cells in the smallest and largest follicles, but in those of intermediate size, the epithelium is pseudostratified columnar.

The cortex of the mature ovary also contains concentrations of fat-filled **vacuolar cells.** Numerous fat vacuoles occur throughout the cytoplasm of these cells, and their nuclei are pyknotic. Collections of these cells are believed to represent regressing postovulatory follicles.

Atretic follicles are commonly found in normal active ovaries. In the most common type of atretic follicle, cells of the membrana granulosa proliferate, forming a number of irregular layers around the oocyte. The oocyte becomes smaller and is eventually replaced by granulosa cells. Ultimately, scar tissue replaces the granulosa cells. In older birds, the oocyte becomes surrounded by hyperplastic and hypertrophied interstitial (luteal) cells during atresia. Both the oocyte and the cells of the membrana granulosa eventually degenerate.

The **oviduct** of the chicken is tortuous and muscular. It consists, in anterioposterior sequence, of the following five regions: **infundibulum, magnum, isthmus, shell gland** (uterus), and **vagina**. From the outside inward, the wall of the oviduct consists of a serosa, muscularis (outer longitudinal and inner circular smooth muscle), lamina propria, and epithelium. In most regions, the lamina propria contains glands.

The infundibulum is composed of a thin-walled funnel and a neck region. Scattered bundles of smooth muscle lie within the connective tissue between the serosa and ciliated, simple columnar epithelium. Longitudinal folds are present in the mucosa within the interior of the funnel near the neck. The folds increase in depth within the neck, and secondary folds appear. The muscularis becomes sorted out into circular and longitudinal layers in the neck.

The magnum is the longest part of the oviduct. Its well developed tubular glands produce albumin. Its mucosal folds are more numerous and taller than those of the infundibulum. Tertiary folds are present. The muscularis is better developed than in the infundibulum. The pseudostratified epithelium is composed of ciliated columnar cells and secretory (goblet) cells.

The isthmus is a relatively short region with a diameter less than that of the magnum. Its longitudinal mucosal folds possess numerous secondary folds. The muscularis is better developed than the magnum's. The epithelium is ciliated, pseudostratified columnar with secretory cells. Its numerous tubular glands secrete the shell membranes.

The uterus is an expanded portion of the oviduct. Its walls are not as thick as those of the preceding segments. The muscularis is well developed, especially the longitudinal layer. The mucosa is thrown into longitudinal, leaf-shaped folds that are covered by a ciliated, pseudostratified, columnar epithelium. The shell of the egg is produced from secretions of its tubular glands.

The vagina is a short, narrow duct. Its muscularis is well developed, especially the circular layer. Its mucosa is thrown into numerous tall, narrow folds bearing many small secondary folds. The surface is covered by a ciliated, pseudostratified columnar epithelium with mucous cells. Sperm storage occurs in the **sperm-host glands**. These tubular glands occur within the connective tissue of the mucosa of the vagina near the junction between the uterus and vagina. After insemination, sperm appear in compact masses within the glands. The vagina of the oviduct opens into the urodeum of the cloaca.

Figure 18.1   ×12.5

Figure 18.2   ×125

Figure 18.3   ×125

Figure 18.4   ×62.5

KEY	
1. Antrum	11. Oocyte, nucleus
2. Corona radiata	12. Primary follicle
3. Corpus luteum	13. Primordial follicles
4. Cortex	14. Stroma
5. Cumulus oophorus	15. Theca externa
6. Granulosa cells	16. Theca folliculi
7. Growing follicles	17. Theca interna
8. Medulla	18. Tunica albuginea
9. Membrana granulosa	19. Zona pellucida
10. Oocyte, cytoplasm	

Figure 18.1. Ovary, Queen. Follicles of various ages and a corpus luteum can be seen in the cortex. A portion of the vascular medulla is present.

Figure 18.2. Ovary, Queen. Early follicles in the outer region of the cortex.

Figure 18.3. Ovary, Bitch. A multilaminar, primary follicle.

Figure 18.4. Ovary, Queen. A young, tertiary follicle.

Figure 18.5

×180

Figure 18.8

×25

Figure 18.5. Ovary, Bitch. Portion of the wall of a tertiary follicle, and part of an adjacent corpus luteum.

Figure 18.6. Corpus Luteum, Ovary, Sow. Peripheral region of a corpus luteum showing theca lutein cells (small) and granulosa lutein cells (large).

Figure 18.7. Ovary, Bitch. Atretic follicles, each with a swollen zona pellucida.

Figure 18.8. Corpus Albicans, Ovary, Cow (Masson's). The scar tissue of the corpus albicans is stained bright blue-green in this preparation.

Figure 18.6

×125

Figure 18.7

×62.5

Figure 18.9   ×62.5

Figure 18.13   ×25

KEY		
1. Corpus luteum	4. Hilus cells	
2. Folds	5. Interstitial gland	
3. Granulosa lutein cell	6. Rete ovarii	

Figure 18.9. Ovary, Bitch. Several interstitial glands are visible within the stroma between two corpora lutea.

Figure 18.10. Interstitial Glands, Ovary, Bitch. Cords of epithelioid cells form the parenchyma of interstitial glands. These glands are well developed in queens and bitches.

Figure 18.11. Hilus Cells, Ovary, Cow. Clusters of epithelioid cells, located in the vicinity of the hilus, are called hilus cells. They resemble the epithelioid cells of the interstitial glands (see Fig. 18.10).

Figure 18.12. Rete Ovarii, Ovary, Cow. Cords of cells, or channels lined by cuboidal epithelial cells, located in the medulla of the ovary are called the rete ovarii. They are considered to be homologous to the rete testis.

Figure 18.13. Fimbria of Infundibulum, Oviduct, Mare. The mucosa of the fimbria is highly folded.

Figure 18.10   ×250

Figure 18.11   ×62.5

Figure 18.12   ×62.5

Figure 18.14 ×125

Figure 18.18 ×12.5

Figure 18.15 ×125

KEY	
1. Adipose tissue, mesosalpinx	6. Lamina propria
2. Cilia	7. Muscularis
3. Columnar epithelium, ciliated	8. Secretory bleb
4. Extruded nucleus	9. Serosa
5. Folds	10. Submucosa

Figure 18.14. Fimbria of Infundibulum, Oviduct, Mare. Detail of the wall. Note the smooth muscle of the thin muscularis.

Figure 18.15. Fimbria of Infundibulum, Oviduct, Cow. Portions of the fimbria may lack smooth muscle, as in this example.

Figure 18.16. Infundibulum, Oviduct, Cow (Masson's). The epithelium consists of ciliated, columnar epithelial cells and nonciliated, secretory cells. Extruded nuclei, which appear to arise from epithelial cells, are common.

Figure 18.17. Infundibulum, Neck, Oviduct, x.s., Cow. The mucosa is highly folded, and the muscularis is thin.

Figure 18.18. Ampulla, Oviduct, x.s., Cow. The mucosa is highly folded. The muscularis is relatively thick. Compare with Figure 18.17.

Figure 18.16 ×250

Figure 18.17 ×12.5

Figure 18.19   ×25

Figure 18.20   ×25

Figure 18.21   ×250

Figure 18.22   ×12.5

Figure 18.23   ×180

KEY	
1. Circular muscle	6. Longitudinal muscle
2. Columnar epithelium	7. Myometrium, circular
3. Cuboidal epithelium	8. Myometrium, longitudinal
4. Endometrial gland	9. Stratum vasculare
5. Folds	

Figure 18.19. Isthmus, Oviduct, x.s., Mare. The mucosa of the isthmus has fewer folds than any other part of the oviduct. The muscularis is thickest in this part of the oviduct.

Figure 18.20. Uterine Horn, x.s., Anestrus, Bitch. The endometrium is thin and the glands are sparse in anestrus.

Figure 18.21. Uterine Horn, x.s., Anestrus, Queen. The lumen of the anestrus uterus is lined by a simple cuboidal epithelium.

Figure 18.22. Uterine Horn, x.s., Proestrus, Bitch. In proestrus, the endometrium becomes thicker and the glands enlarge.

Figure 18.23. Uterine Horn, x.s., Proestrus, Bitch. Luminal epithelial cells become columnar during proestrus and estrus.

Figure 18.24 ×12.5

Figure 18.28 ×250

Figure 18.25 ×12.5

KEY	
1. Artery	7. Stratum vasculare
2. Endometrial gland	8. Tunica adventitia
3. Mesometrium	9. Tunica intima
4. Myometrium	10. Tunica media
5. Myometrium, circular	11. Vein
6. Myometrium, longitudinal	

Figure 18.24. Uterine Horn, x.s., Estrus, Bitch. A thick endometrium and highly developed glands are characteristic of the estrous uterus.

Figure 18.25. Uterine Horn, x.s., Diestrus, Bitch. The endometrium and its glands become fully developed during diestrus.

Figure 18.26. Mesometrium, Bitch. The mesometrium contains an abundance of smooth muscle and numerous blood vessels. Smooth muscle of the mesometrium is continuous with the outer, longitudinal layer of the myometrium.

Figure 18.27. Uterine Horn, Brood Mare (Orcein). There is an abundance of elastic fibers (red-brown in this micrograph) in the intima and adventitia of blood vessels of the uterus of animals that have been through a pregnancy. The section is from the midregion of the myometrium.

Figure 18.28. Uterine Horn, Brood Mare. Detail of a portion of an artery in the myometrium. The intima becomes thickened with elastic fibers and smooth muscle in animals who have experienced a pregnancy. The adventitia also becomes heavily infiltrated with elastic fibers.

Figure 18.26 ×12.5

Figure 18.27 ×25

Figure 18.29

×25

Figure 18.30

×125

Figure 18.31

×250

Figure 18.32

×12.5

Figure 18.33

×180

KEY	
1. Blood vessels	6. Hemorrhagic region
2. Caruncle	7. Myometrium, circular
3. Cilia	8. Myometrium, longitudinal
4. Cuboidal epithelium	9. Pseudostratified epithelium
5. Endometrial gland	

Figure 18.29. Uterine Horn, x.s., Metestrus, Cow. Metestrous bleeding occurs in the cow. Numerous erythrocytes of hemorrhagic regions can be seen beneath the surface epithelium (see Fig. 18.30).

Figure 18.30. Uterus, Metestrus, Cow. Detail of Figure 18.29. Hemorrhagic regions are evident in the endometrium beneath the surface epithelium. The epithelial cells are cuboidal during metestrus in the cow.

Figure 18.31. Uterine Horn, Cow (Masson's). The epithelial cells lining the uterine glands are sometimes ciliated, as in this section.

Figure 18.32. Caruncle, Uterus, x.s., Cow. The endometrium of the uterus of ruminants contains nonglandular, highly cellular prominences called caruncles. Uterine glands that lie deep to the caruncle open near its base.

Figure 18.33. Caruncle, Uterus, Cow. The caruncle consists of highly cellular (mostly fibroblasts) connective tissue, and numerous blood vessels located beneath the epithelium.

Figure 18.34

Figure 18.35 ×25

Figure 18.36 ×62.5

KEY	
1. Allantoic blood vessel	6. Marginal hematoma
2. Allantoic epithelium	7. Myometrium
3. Chorioallantoic membrane	8. Placental labyrinth
4. Chorion laeve	9. Spongy layer
5. Deep glandular layer	10. Supraglandular layer

Figure 18.34. Placenta (Zonary and Endotheliochorial), Bitch (Drawing). Carnivores have a zonary placenta that appears, grossly, as a beltlike band around the middle of the chorionic sac. The chorionic (fetal) tissue penetrates to the endothelium of the maternal blood vessels. A placenta with this type of fetal-maternal junction is called an endotheliochorial placenta. The association between the maternal endothelium and syntrophoblast can be seen in Figures 18.37 and 18.39.

Note: This drawing is of a section through a portion of one of the edges of the zonary placenta of a bitch.

Figure 18.35. Placenta (Zonary and Endotheliochorial), Bitch (Trichrome). Section through the deepest layers of the placenta (see Fig. 18.34 for location). The spongy layer is formed by the occluded uterine glands in the mid-region of the endometrium. The deep glandular layer consists of the bases of the uterine glands. The supraglandular layer is a sheet of connective tissue between the deep glandular and spongy layers. (Photomicrograph of a histologic section borrowed from the College of Veterinary Medicine, Iowa State University.)

Figure 18.36. Placenta (Zonary and Endotheliochorial), Bitch (Trichrome). Portion of the chorioallantoic membrane and the placental labyrinth (see Fig. 18.34 for location). The chorioallantoic membrane in this micrograph appears thicker than normal because of the presence of extensive space artifact. Note the presence of fetal blood vessels in the chorioallantoic membrane. (Photomicrograph of a histologic section borrowed from the College of Veterinary Medicine, Iowa State University.)

Figure 18.37

×125

Figure 18.38

×250

Figure 18.39

×62.5

Figure 18.40

×125

Figure 18.37. Placenta (Zonary and Endotheliochorial), Bitch (Trichrome). Section is through the placental labyrinth. Both maternal and fetal components of this endotheliochorial placenta can be seen. (Photomicrograph of a histologic section borrowed from the College of Veterinary Medicine, Iowa State University.)

Figure 18.38. Placenta (Zonary and Endotheliochorial), Bitch (Trichrome). Detail of the placental labyrinth. The maternal blood vessels are lined by endothelial cells with bulging nuclei. (Photomicrograph of a histologic section borrowed from the College of Veterinary Medicine, Iowa State University.)

Figure 18.39. Placenta (Zonary and Endotheliochorial), Bitch (Trichrome). Trophoblastic projections, lined by large, pale, vacuolated cells, protrude into spaces (areolae) in the region where the placental labyrinth is forming. A portion of the maternal tissue, which has been partially destroyed by the invading trophoblast, is represented by the red-stained, necrotic tissue seen in the lower left quadrant of the micrograph. (Photomicrograph of a histologic section borrowed from the College of Veterinary Medicine, Iowa State University.)

Figure 18.40. Placenta (Zonary and Endotheliochorial), Bitch (Trichrome). Detail of Figure 18.39. (Photomicrograph of a histologic section borrowed from the College of Veterinary Medicine, Iowa State University.)

Figure 18.41   ×12.5

Figure 18.41. Placenta (Zonary and Endotheliochorial), Bitch (Trichrome). A portion of a marginal hematoma, consisting of large compartments filled with blood derived from hemorrhaging uterine blood vessels, is shown (see Fig. 18.34 for location). (Photomicrograph of a histologic section borrowed from the College of Veterinary Medicine, Iowa State University.)

Figure 18.42. Chorion Laeve, Bitch (Trichrome). The chorion laeve is the part of the chorioallantoic sac that is not involved in the formation of the placenta. Its surface is smooth and is apposed to the uterine epithelium. This section is from the region adjacent to the hematoma of the placenta (see Fig. 18.34 for location). (Photomicrograph of a histologic section borrowed from the College of Veterinary Medicine, Iowa State University.)

Figure 18.43. Placenta (Diffuse and Epitheliochorial), Mare. In the horse small tufts of branched chorioallantoic villi interdigitate with crypts of the endometrium. Together, the tufts and the crypts form structures called microplacentomes. (Photomicrograph of a histologic section borrowed from the College of Veterinary Medicine, Iowa State University.)

Figure 18.44. Placenta (Diffuse and Epitheliochorial), Mare. Detail of a microplacentome. Longitudinal and cross sections of chorioallantoic villi are surrounded by endometrial crypts. The epithelium of the crypts, which may vary in height, is flattened in this region. The villi contain blood vessels and connective tissue and are covered by pink-stained trophoblast cells. (Photomicrograph of a histologic section borrowed from the College of Veterinary Medicine, Iowa State University.)

Figure 18.42   ×62.5

Figure 18.43   ×25

Figure 18.44   ×125

Figure 18.45   ×125

Figure 18.46   ×12.5

Figure 18.47   ×180

Figure 18.48   ×12.5

KEY	
1. Allantoic blood vessel	10. Endometrium, secondary fold
2. Chorioallantoic membrane	11. High columnar cells
3. Chorioallantoic membrane, primary fold	12. Intercotyledonary endometrium
4. Chorioallantoic membrane, secondary fold	13. Low columnar cells
5. Chorioallantoic villus, epithelium	14. Maternal blood vessel
6. Crypt, epithelium	15. Myometrium
7. Cuboidal cells	16. Placentome
8. Endometrium, connective tissue	17. Space artifact
9. Endometrium, primary fold	18. Stalk of placentome
	19. Uterine gland

Figure 18.45. Placenta (Diffuse and Epitheliochorial), Mare. Detail of a placentome adjacent to the endometrium. The epithelium of the endometrial crypt consists of pale, cuboidal cells. The epithelium of the chorioallantoic villi is formed from pink-stained cuboidal and low columnar cells. (Photomicrograph of a histologic section borrowed from the College of Veterinary Medicine, Iowa State University.)

Figure 18.46. Placenta (Diffuse and Epitheliochorial), Sow (Trichrome). The placenta of the sow is folded, diffuse, and epitheliochorial. Folds of the chorioallantoic membrane interdigitate with folds of the uterus. (Photomicrograph of a histologic section borrowed from the College of Veterinary Medicine, Iowa State University.)

Figure 18.47. Placenta (Diffuse and Epitheliochorial), Sow (Trichrome). Interdigitating secondary folds of the chorioallantoic membrane and endometrium. The bases of the folds of the chorioallantoic membrane are lined by high columnar epithelial cells, whereas the crests of the maternal folds are covered by shorter columnar cells. The remainder of both epithelial surfaces is lined by cuboidal or flattened cells. Note that the chorioallantoic epithelial surface is invaded by capillaries. (Photomicrograph of a histologic section borrowed from the College of Veterinary Medicine, Iowa State University.)

Figure 18.48. Placenta (Cotyledonary and Epitheliochorial), Cow. A section through a placentome formed from the association of a cotyledon (clumps of chorioallantoic villi) with a uterine caruncle (endometrial elevation). Note that the endometrial epithelium of the intercotyledonary region is discontinuous.

Figure 18.49 ×25

Figure 18.53 ×250

Figure 18.50 ×125

KEY	
1. Allantoic blood vessel	8. Lamina propria
2. Chorioallantoic villus, branch	9. Primary fold
3. Chorioallantoic villus, main stem	10. Secondary fold
4. Cilia	11. Stratified squamous
5. Crypt	epithelium
6. Cryptal epithelium	12. Tertiary fold
7. Diplokaryocyte	

Figure 18.49. Placenta (Cotyledonary and Epitheliochorial), Cow. Detail of Figure 18.48. Highly branched chorioallantoic villi interdigitate with uterine crypts.

Figure 18.50. Placenta (Cotyledonary and Epitheliochorial), Cow. Detail of a portion of a placentome adjacent to the stalk. Note that the cryptal epithelium is cuboidal or flattened. The epithelium of the chorioallantoic villus consists of irregularly shaped cells and binucleate giant cells (diplokaryocytes).

Figure 18.51. Cervix of Uterus, Bitch. The mucosa of the cervix is thrown into folds. The epithelium of the bitch's cervix is stratified squamous. (Photomicrograph of a histologic section borrowed from the College of Veterinary Medicine, Iowa State University.)

Figure 18.52. Cervix of Uterus, Mare. Cervical folds are evident.

Figure 18.53. Cervix of Uterus, Mare (Masson's). The cervical epithelium is simple columnar, except in the bitch (see Fig. 18.51). Epithelial cells may be ciliated.

Figure 18.51 ×125

Figure 18.52 ×12.5

Figure 18.54   ×125

Figure 18.58   ×62.5

Figure 18.55   ×62.5

KEY	
1. Adventitia	8. Muscularis
2. Cavernous spaces	9. Stratified epithelium
3. Columnar cells	10. Stratified squamous epithe-
4. Duct	lium
5. Keratinized cells	11. Transitional epithelium
6. Lamina propria	12. Urethral epithelium
7. Minor vestibular gland	13. Vestibular epithelium

Figure 18.54. Vagina, Anestrus, Bitch. The epithelium of the carnivore's anestrous vagina is stratified squamous to stratified cuboidal. (Photomicrograph of a histologic section borrowed from the College of Veterinary Medicine, Iowa State University.)

Figure 18.55. Vagina, Estrus, Queen. In carnivores, the vagina is lined by a thickened, keratinized, stratified squamous epithelium during estrus. Exfoliated keratinized cells are visible in the vaginal lumen in this micrograph.

Figure 18.56. Urethra, x.s., Queen. Section was taken from the region close to the bladder. This portion of the urethra is lined by a transitional epithelium. (Photomicrograph of a histologic section borrowed from the College of Veterinary Medicine, Iowa State University.)

Figure 18.56   ×62.5

Figure 18.57. Junction of Vestibule and Urethra, x.s., Queen. Near the vestibule, the urethra is lined by a stratified squamous epithelium. Note the presence of cavernous spaces in the connective tissue adjacent to the muscularis. Such spaces occur only in the distal two-thirds of the urethra in the doe, ewe, and queen. In all other domestic mammals, cavernous spaces occur throughout the entire length of the urethra.

Figure 18.58. Vestibule, Queen. Detail of a minor vestibular gland. The secretory tubules of these branched, tubular glands are lined by columnar cells. Their ducts are lined by stratified squamous epithelium.

Figure 18.57   ×12.5

Figure 18.59 ×62.5

Figure 18.63 ×125

KEY	
1. Columnar cells	5. Neutrophil
2. Duct	6. Parabasal cell
3. Erythrocyte	7. Superficial cell
4. Intermediate cell	8. Superficial intermediate cell

Figure 18.59. Vestibule, Queen. Detail of a major vestibular gland. These glands are found in queens and ruminants. They are compound tubular glands with secretory units like those of the minor vestibular glands (see Fig. 18.58).

Figure 18.60. Vaginal Smear, Anestrus, Bitch (Hema-3). During anestrus, parabasal and intermediate cells are the predominant epithelial cells present (see introduction for description of cell types). Neutrophils and bacteria may be present in limited numbers.

Figure 18.61. Vaginal Smear, Early Proestrus, Bitch (Hema-3). During early to mid proestrus, smears may contain neutrophils, erythrocytes, and various epithelial-cell types (parabasal, intermediate, superficial intermediate, and superficial cells).

Figure 18.62. Vaginal Smear, Mid to Late Proestrus, Bitch (Diff-Quik). In late proestrus, superficial intermediate and superficial cells are predominant. Neutrophils decrease in number at this time.

Figure 18.63. Vaginal Smear, Estrus, Bitch (Diff-Quik). Most (90% or more) of the epithelial cells from a bitch in estrus are superficial cells. Erythrocytes may be present in small numbers. Some estrous smears may contain large numbers of bacteria. Neutrophils are not normally present.

Figure 18.60 ×125

Figure 18.61 ×125

Figure 18.62 ×125

Figure 18.64   ×125

Figure 18.65   ×12.5

Figure 18.66   ×62.5

Figure 18.67   ×250

Figure 18.68   ×62.5

KEY	
1. Follicle, early	8. Oocyte, nucleus
2. Follicle, late	9. Oocyte, yolk-laden cytoplasm
3. Granulocytes	10. Parabasal cell
4. Intermediate cell	11. Superficial cell
5. Medulla	12. Superficial intermediate cell
6. Neutrophil	13. Vacuolar cells
7. Oocyte	

Figure 18.64. Vaginal Smear, Diestrus, Bitch (Diff-Quik). There is a significant change in the numbers of epithelial-cell types during diestrus. Superficial cells decrease, and parabasal and intermediate cells increase. Neutrophils usually reappear during diestrus. Because erythrocytes may be present in smears from bitches in early diestrus, it is not possible to distinguish proestrus from diestrus on the basis of a single smear.

Figure 18.65. Ovary, Hen. A portion of the ovarian cortex with developing follicles.

Figure 18.66. Ovary, Vacuolar Cells, Hen. A portion of the cortex with a mass of fat-laden vacuolar cells. The latter may represent regressing postovulatory follicles.

Figure 18.67. Ovary, Vacuolar Cells, Hen. Detail of Figure 18.66. Vacuolar cells have pyknotic nuclei and contain numerous fat vacuoles. Cell boundaries are often indistinct.

Figure 18.68. Ovary, Granulocytes, Hen. Granulocytes are often found in the cortex of mature ovaries. The acidophilic granules of these cells impart a red tinge to a large area of the cortex in this micrograph.

Figure 18.69   ×250

Figure 18.73

Figure 18.70   ×25

Figure 18.69. Ovary, Developing Follicle, Hen. A portion of the wall of a developing follicle. Note the flattened cells of the theca interna and the presence of interstitial cells in the theca externa.

Figure 18.70. Ovary, Atretic Follicle, Hen. In some atretic follicles, interstitial (luteal) cells proliferate, hypertrophy, and migrate inward (see Fig. 18.71).

Figure 18.71. Ovary, Atretic Follicle, Hen. Detail of Figure 18.70.

Figure 18.72. Ovary, Atretic Follicle, Hen. Cells of the membrana granulosa have proliferated, forming a thick layer characteristic of many atretic follicles.

Figure 18.73. Oviduct, Diagrammatic Drawing, Hen. The oviduct of the hen is divisible into an infundibulum, magnum, isthmus, uterus, and vagina.

Figure 18.71   ×125

Figure 18.72   ×12.5

Figure 18.74   ×62.5

Figure 18.75   ×62.5

Figure 18.76   ×250

Figure 18.77   ×12.5

Figure 18.78   ×25

KEY	
1. Ciliated epithelium	10. Pseudostratified columnar epithelium
2. Glandular groove	11. Regenerating gland
3. Lamina propria	12. Resting gland
4. Mucosa	13. Secondary fold
5. Mucosal fold, infundibulum	14. Secretory gland
6. Mucosal fold, magnum	15. Serosa
7. Muscularis	16. Tertiary fold
8. Muscularis, circular	
9. Primary fold	

Figure 18.74. Funnel of Infundibulum, Oviduct, x.s., Hen. The mucosa is thrown into shallow ridges that increase in height as the funnel narrows toward the neck region. The epithelium is ciliated, simple columnar. Scattered bundles of smooth muscle form the muscularis. A serosa covers the funnel externally.

Figure 18.75. Neck of Infundibulum, x.s., Oviduct, Hen. Tall primary mucosal folds bear secondary and tertiary folds.

Figure 18.76. Neck of Infundibulum, x.s., Oviduct, Hen. Detail of mucosa showing folds lined by ciliated columnar cells. The bottoms of the grooves between the folds are lined by nonciliated secretory cells.

Figure 18.77. Neck of Infundibulum and Magnum, x.s., Oviduct, Hen. The primary mucosal folds of the magnum are taller and broader vis-à-vis the infundibulum, because of the presence of numerous tubular glands.

Figure 18.78. Magnum, x.s., Oviduct, Hen. Portion of a fold. Depending on their activity, the tubular glands of the magnum exhibit distinctive features. Three morphologic phases of activity can be recognized (regenerating, secretory, resting) (see Figs. 18.80 and 18.81 for details).

Figure 18.79 ×250

Figure 18.83 ×125

Figure 18.80 ×250

KEY	
1. Albumen	6. Isthmus, primary fold
2. Ciliated cell	7. Magnum
3. Epithelium, regenerating gland	8. Muscularis
	9. Pseudostratified epithelium
4. Epithelium, resting gland	10. Secretory cell
5. Epithelium, secretory gland	11. Tubular gland

Figure 18.79. Magnum, Oviduct, Hen. Detail of the epithelium. Ciliated columnar and secretory (goblet) cells comprise the epithelium of the magnum. The nuclei of the secretory cells are round and are located close to the base of the cell, whereas the nuclei of the ciliated cells are oval and occupy the central to apical region of the cell. Accordingly, the epithelium is pseudostratified columnar.

Figure 18.80. Magnum, Oviduct, Hen. Detail of regenerating tubular glands. These glands have clearly defined lumens. The secretory cells are cuboidal.

Figure 18.81 ×250

Figure 18.81. Magnum, Oviduct, Hen. Detail of secretory tubular glands and resting tubular glands. The cells of the secretory stage are characterized by pyknotic, basal nuclei. The entire cytoplasm is filled with strongly acidophilic granules. The glandular lumens may be dilated by secreted albumen. The cytoplasm of the cells in the resting stage has a frothy appearance, and the lumens of the glands are obscure.

Figure 18.82. Isthmus, x.s., Oviduct, Hen. The primary folds of the isthmus are not as broad as those of the magnum. Compare with figure 18.77. They are somewhat angular in appearance. A portion of an adjacent region of the magnum is present in this micrograph.

Figure 18.83. Isthmus, Oviduct, Hen. A portion of the epithelium and underlying tubular glands. The epithelium is ciliated pseudostratified columnar. A tubular gland can be seen opening to the surface. The glandular cells do not undergo obvious cyclic changes as in the magnum.

Figure 18.82 ×12.5

Figure 18.84 ×12.5

Figure 18.88 ×125

Figure 18.85 ×250

Figure 18.86 ×625

KEY	
1. Apical cell	8. Muscularis
2. Basal cell, nucleus	9. Primary fold
3. Blood vessel	10. Pseudostratified epithelium
4. Concave surface	11. Secondary fold
5. Duct	12. Sperm-host gland
6. Erythrocyte in capillary	13. Vacuole
7. Glandular epithelium	

Figure 18.84. Uterus (Shell Gland), Oviduct, Hen. The folds of the uterus are not as broad as those of the magnum, and there is less glandular tissue. This section was taken from a uterus that had been fixed while containing an egg. Accordingly, the luminal surface is somewhat concave.

Figure 18.85. Uterus (Shell Gland), Oviduct, Hen. Ducts of complex, branched, tubular glands pierce the ciliated pseudostratified columnar epithelium at intervals. Ducts are formed from polygonal gland cells.

Figure 18.86. Uterus (Shell Gland), Oviduct, Hen. Basal cells (nuclei close to the basement membrane) of the pseudostratified epithelium may contain vacuoles above and below their nuclei. Apical cells (nuclei centrally located) contain numerous granules before releasing their secretion.

Figure 18.87. Vagina, x.s., Oviduct, Hen. The mucosa of the vagina is characterized by long, slender, primary folds bearing numerous small secondary folds. The muscularis is highly developed.

Figure 18.88. Vagina, Proximal, Oviduct, Hen. Sperm-host glands are tubular glands, lined by tall columnar cells, and are located within the mucosa of the vagina near the uterovaginal junction. Sperm are stored in these glands, remaining functional for up to 21 days.

Figure 18.87 ×25

19

THE EYE

MAMMALS

The eye is a sensory organ designed for vision. Basically, it is composed of a **lens** and a wall that is divided into three layers: an outer **fibrous tunic** (corneoscleral layer), a middle **vascular tunic** (uvea), and an inner **retinal tunic**. The fibrous tunic is divided into the posterior, opaque sclera and the anterior, transparent cornea. The vascular tunic includes the choroid, ciliary body, and iris. The retinal tunic consists of a ten-layered, photosensitive retina and a bilayered, nonphotosensitive portion that covers the ciliary body and the posterior surface of the iris.

The eye contains three fluid-filled regions. The **anterior chamber** is bordered by the cornea, iris, and lens. The **posterior chamber** is located between the iris, lens, zonular fibers, and ciliary processes. Both of these chambers contain aqueous humor. The most posterior compartment, the **cavity of the vitreous humor,** lies behind the lens.

The transparent, biconvex **lens** is avascular. It is composed entirely of epithelial cells enclosed within a homogeneous capsule. The cells on the anterior surface of the lens just below the capsule are simple cuboidal and form the **lens epithelium.** Toward the equator of the lens, the cells become long, prismatic, and arranged in meridional rows, forming **lens fibers.** As new lens fibers develop from the lens epithelium at the germinal zone of the equator, older lens fibers are displaced centrally and lose their nuclei. The lens is suspended by **zonular fibers** that extend from the lens capsule to the ciliary processes.

The **sclera** consists of densely interwoven bundles of collagenous fibers arranged parallel to the surface of the wall of the eye. There are also fibroblasts, some fine elastic fibers, and scattered melanocytes, especially in the innermost region of the sclera.

The **cornea** is avascular. Its anterior (outer) surface is covered by the nonkeratinized, stratified squamous **anterior epithelium.** Below this layer is **Bowman's membrane,** which is not distinct in domestic mammals. The underlying **stroma** (substantia propria) is composed of thin lamellae of collagenous fibers oriented parallel to the corneal surface. Fibroblasts occur between the layers of fibers. **Descemet's membrane** is a relatively thick membrane that separates the stroma from the **posterior epithelium.** The latter consists of a single layer of squamous to low cuboidal cells that covers the posterior surface of the cornea.

The corneoscleral junction is called the **limbus**. Here, the regular collagenous lamellae of the corneal stroma merge with the interwoven fibers of the sclera. The appearance of the stratified squamous epithelium of the cornea differs from that of the bulbar conjunctiva, which overlies the sclera near the limbus. The deepest cells in the epithelium of the bulbar conjunctiva are smaller and more closely packed than those of the anterior epithelium of the cornea. In addition, the basal border of the conjunctival epithelium is uneven with the presence of an underlying, papillated layer of loose connective tissue. The boundary between the corneal epithelium and its underlying stroma, however, is smooth.

The **choroid** is the portion of the vascular tunic of the eye that lies between the sclera and the photosensitive retina. It contains numerous melanocytes. The fine network of connective tissue of the **suprachoroid layer** joins the sclera to the **vascular layer** of the choroid. The latter is composed of a profusion of blood vessels surrounded by loose connective tissue. The **choriocapillary layer** contains a thin network of capillaries that are distributed in a single plane. **Bruch's membrane,** a refractile membrane that lies between the choriocapillary layer and the pigment epithelium of the retina, is difficult to resolve.

A reflective **tapetum lucidum** is located between the choriocapillary and vascular layers of the choroid in the dorsal portion of the eye. It is present in all domestic mammals except the pig. The horse and ruminants have a **fibrous tapetum lucidum** composed of layers of collagenous fibers and fibroblasts. The cat and dog have a **cellular tapetum lucidum** formed by flattened, pentagonal or hexagonal cells that appear bricklike in profile. The tapetal cells are filled with numerous rod-shaped granules. The flat surfaces of the cells and the long axes of their rod-shaped granules lie parallel to the surface of the retina.

The **ciliary body** is an anterior continuation of the choroid that extends to the base of the iris. The loose connective tissue of the stroma contains smooth muscle, the **ciliary muscle,** that lies peripheral to an inner, vascular region. The epithelium of the ciliary body, which is formed by cells of the nonphotosensitive portion of the retina, is called the **pars ciliaris retinae**. It is a bilayer of cells consisting of a basal layer of pigmented cells and a surface layer of nonpigmented columnar cells. Short folds of the posterior surface of the ciliary body become longer toward the iris and form **ciliary processes** that project toward the lens. Zonular fibers extend from the processes to the lens capsule near the equator of the lens.

The **iris** is the most anterior part of the uveal tract. It forms a thin, contractile diaphragm with a central aperature, the **pupil**. The base of the iris is attached to the anterior portion of the ciliary body. The **stroma** of connective tissue of the iris contains many melanocytes and blood vessels. The stroma contains circumferentially arranged bundles of smooth muscle that form the **sphincter** (constrictor) **muscle.** The anterior surface of the iris is not covered by an epithelium, but rather by a discontinuous layer of stromal cells (fibroblasts and melanocytes). The posterior surface is covered by a bilayer of epithelial cells, the **pars iridica retinae,** which represents the most anterior continuation of the nonphotosensitive portion of the retina. It consists of a superficial layer of **pigmented columnar cells** and a basal layer of partially **pigmented myoepithelial cells**. The latter are elongated, radially arranged, contractile cells that form the dilator "muscle" of the iris. They have an apical, pigmented portion containing the nucleus and a nonpigmented basal portion. The nonpigmented regions of these cells border the stroma and appear as an acidophilic band. The pigmented portion of each myoepithelial cell lies just below the layer of pigmented columnar cells. In the horse, pig, and ruminant a number of **corpora nigra** (iris granules) project from the pupillary margin of the iris. They are highly vascularized proliferations of the stroma and the pigmented epithelial cells of the iris.

At the peripheral margin of the anterior chamber is the **filtration angle,** the area between the limbus, the base of the iris, and the ciliary body. This triangular region is spanned by a latticework of trabeculae and intertrabecular, fluid-filled spaces. The trabeculae are composed of connective tissue and pigment cells and are covered by a single layer of squamous cells. They form the **pectinate ligament,** the **uveal trabecular meshwork,** and the **corneoscleral trabecular meshwork.** At the peripheral margin of the anterior chamber, excess aqueous humor passes through the openings within the pectinate ligament into the **spaces of Fontana** within the uveal trabecular meshwork. These spaces communicate with those of the corneoscleral trabecular meshwork, which drain into the **scleral venous plexus.** In the horse the limbus does not overlap the pectinate ligament of the filtration angle, so that the pectinate ligament is apparent by direct examination of the eye. In the other domestic mammals the limbus covers the pectinate ligament, which is therefore obscured from view by the opaque sclera.

The **retina** is the innermost layer of the wall of the eye. The photosensitive portion lines the inner surface of the eye (adjacent to the cavity of the vitreous humor) from the **ora ciliaris retinae** to the optic disc. The latter is the point of transition from the photosensitive retina to the nonphotosensitive retina. From the ora ciliaris retinae, the nonphotosensitive portion continues anteriorly as a bilayer of cells, forming the pars ciliaris retinae and the pars iridica retinae, which cover the ciliary body and the posterior surface of the iris, respectively.

From the choroid to the cavity of the vitreous humor, the 10 layers of the photosensitive retina are as follows:

Pigment epithelium
Layer of rods and cones
Outer limiting membrane (usually not apparent)
Outer nuclear layer
Outer plexiform layer
Inner nuclear layer
Inner plexiform layer
Ganglion cell layer
Nerve fiber layer
Inner limiting membrane

In that part of the eye where the tapetum lucidum is located, the cuboidal cells of the pigment epithelium contain few or no pigment granules. In other parts of the eye, pigment granules are numerous in the cells of the pigment epithelium.

The nerve-fiber layer consists of axonal processes of the ganglion cells that converge at the **optic disc** and form the optic nerve. Because photoreceptor cells are not present here, this region is also referred to as the blind spot. Bundles of fibers of the optic nerve pass through perforations of the sclera. This sievelike part of the sclera is the **lamina cribrosa**.

The **conjunctiva** is a thin, transparent, mucous membrane. The **bulbar conjunctiva** is continuous with the anterior surface of the cornea at the limbus and covers the sclera for a short distance. The **palpebral conjunctiva** lines the internal surface of the eyelids. The **fornix of the conjunctiva** is the point of reflexion of the bulbar and palpebral conjunctiva. The epithelium of the conjunctiva varies from stratified squamous to stratified columnar and may even appear transitional. Goblet cells are often present. The underlying layer of loose connective tissue may contain diffuse or nodular lymphatic tissue.

The **eyelids** are covered internally by the palpebral conjunctiva and externally by thin skin. The skin contains hair follicles, sweat glands (glands of Moll), and sebaceous glands (glands of Zeiss). In the pig the glands are particularly well developed. Between the dermis of the skin and the lamina propria of the palpebral conjunctiva is a plate of dense connective tissue, the **tarsus** (tarsal plate). Large, multilobular, sebaceous glands, called **tarsal (Meibomian) glands,** are embedded in the tarsus. Their central ducts open onto the palpebral surface near its junction with the skin.

The **nictitating membrane** (third eyelid) is a ventromedial fold of conjunctiva. It is supported by hyaline cartilage in the dog and ruminants and by elastic cartilage in the cat, horse, and pig. The **superficial gland of the nictitating membrane** surrounds the base of the cartilage. It is a serous gland in the horse and cat, mixed in the dog and ruminants, and mucous in the pig. The pig also has a **Harderian gland** (deep gland of the nictitating membrane) that produces a fatty secretion.

The **lacrimal gland** is a tubuloacinar gland, serous in the cat and mixed in the horse, ruminant, dog, and pig. It is predominantly a mucous gland in the pig and mostly serous in the horse and ruminant. There are also accessory lacrimal glands, such as Krause's gland, which may be serous or mixed.

CHICKEN

The eye of the chicken is quite different from that of mammals. Within the **capsule** the **lens** is divided into the **annular pad** and the **lens body.** The annular pad forms an outer ring around the equator of the lens body. It consists of radially arranged lens fibers with peripheral nuclei. In the lens body the lens fibers are oriented parallel to the optical axis of the eye, and some nuclei are present, primarily near the annular pad.

A remarkable feature of the avian **sclera** is the presence of a ring of overlapping **scleral ossicles,** anteriorly, and a cup-shaped layer of hyaline cartilage, the **scleral cartilage,** posteriorly. The latter terminates internal to the scleral ossicles. Dense connective tissue encloses the scleral ossicles and extends posteriorly, peripheral to the cartilage layer.

The layers of the **cornea** of the chicken are similar to those of mammals. Bowman's membrane, however, is thicker and therefore more apparent in histologic preparations. Descemet's membrane is relatively thin and less distinct.

The **choroid** is a thick, vascularized coat with numerous pigment cells. The suprachoroid abuts the thin perichondrium of the scleral cartilage. The vascular layer of the choroid contains blood vessels and large spaces embedded in loose connective tissue. The choriocapillary layer is separated from the pigment epithelium of the retina by an indistinct Bruch's membrane. No tapetum lucidum is present in the chicken.

The **ciliary body** is a thin layer of loose connective tissue with a thick outer region of numerous elastic fibers. It is covered by a bilayer of more or less cuboidal, pigmented basal cells and cuboidal to columnar, nonpigmented surface cells. Folds of the lining of the ciliary body form ciliary processes that fuse to the lens capsule in the region of the equator of the lens. More posteriorly, zonular fibers extend from the ciliary body to the lens capsule. The ciliary muscles (Crampton's and Brücke's) are skeletal muscles that lie across from the ciliary body, just inside the main portion of the sclera.

The **iris** is thickest just above its narrow base, then tapers toward the pupillary margin. The stroma contains a sphincter and dilator muscle. Both of these are formed from small skeletal muscle cells that contain lipid vacuoles. The dilator muscle is sparse and posterior to the thicker sphincter muscle. The anterior (corneal) surface of the iris is covered by a simple layer of nonpigmented, flattened epithelial cells. The posterior (lens) surface of the iris is covered by a stratified layer of pigmented epithelial cells, three to five cells thick.

The photosensitive **retina** of the chicken is composed of 10 layers, as in mammals, but unlike that in mammals is avascular. The cells of the pigment epithelium are considerably different in the chicken. They are tall and narrow rather than cuboidal. The nucleus occupies the smaller, basal region of each cell, which contains few or no pigment granules. The apical portion is filled with rod-shaped pigment granules that are oriented parallel to the long axis of the cell. The apical cytoplasm often appears to be separated into tufts or strands of pigment granules.

The **pecten** is a thin, highly vascular, pleated membrane that protrudes into the cavity of the vitreous humor from the ventral surface of the eye. Its base is secured intermittently to the linear, optic disc. The apical surface is attached to a thickened mass of pectineal tissue called the **bridge.** The pecten is characterized by an extensive network of capillaries lined by thick endothelial cells with plump nuclei. Polymorphic pigment cells fill the spaces between the capillaries and larger vessels. The pecten is draped by a **covering membrane,** which is thought to be continuous with the inner limiting membrane of the retina.

The **filtration angle** of the chicken is somewhat different from that of mammals. It is filled by a trabecular meshwork formed by the **pectinate ligament** (uveal meshwork) and the **scleral trabecular meshwork**. The pectinate ligament is a loose network of elastic fibers covered by simple squamous cells. It spans the filtration angle from the scleral trabecular meshwork to the iris and the elastic tissue of the ciliary body. The trabecular meshwork of the pectinate ligament encloses the **spaces of Fontana**. The latter communicate with the spaces of the scleral trabecular meshwork, which is formed by collagenous and elastic fibers. These spaces communicate with the **canal of Schlemm** within the sclera.

The chicken has a thin, well-developed **nictitating** membrane. A supportive cartilage is absent. The inner surface of the **eyelids** is lined by the palpebral conjunctiva. The external surface is covered by thin skin with sparse feathers. No glands are present.

The **lacrimal gland** is a small, tubular gland that produces a mucous secretion. It lies medial to the caudal part of the lower eyelid. The **Harderian gland** is a larger gland that lies on the dorsal posterior surface of the eye. It is characterized by numerous plasma cells that surround the tubular secretory units.

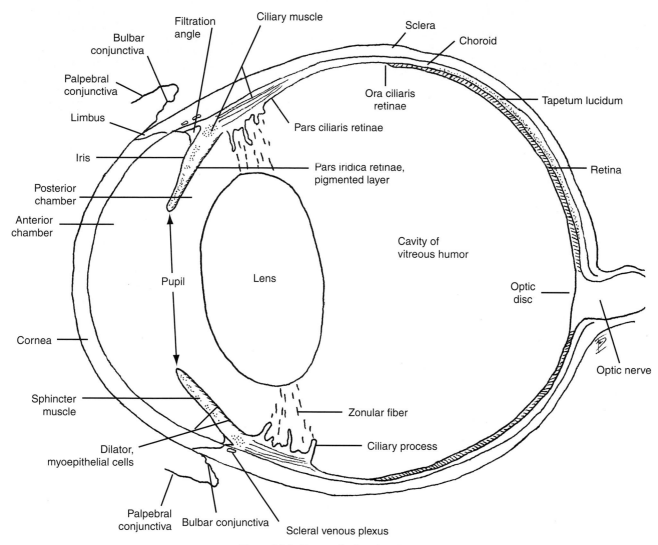

Bulbar conjunctiva

Palpebral conjunctiva

Limbus

Iris

Posterior chamber

Anterior chamber

Cornea

Sphincter muscle

Dilator, myoepithelial cells

Filtration angle

Ciliary muscle

Sclera

Choroid

Ora ciliaris retinae

Pars ciliaris retinae

Tapetum lucidum

Pars iridica retinae, pigmented layer

Retina

Pupil

Lens

Cavity of vitreous humor

Optic disc

Optic nerve

Zonular fiber

Ciliary process

Palpebral conjunctiva

Bulbar conjunctiva

Scleral venous plexus

Figure 19.1. Eye, sagittal section, Dog.

Figure 19.2 ×12.5

Figure 19.3 ×125

Figure 19.4 ×125

Figure 19.5 ×250

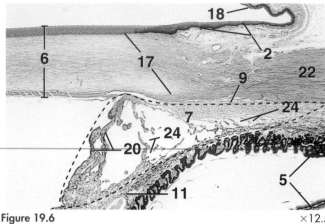

Figure 19.6 ×12.5

KEY	
1. Anterior chamber	13. Lens capsule
2. Bulbar conjunctiva	14. Lens epithelium
3. Ciliary body	15. Lens fibers, new
4. Ciliary muscle	16. Lens fibers, old
5. Ciliary process	17. Limbus
6. Cornea	18. Palpebral conjunctiva
7. Corneoscleral trabecular meshwork	19. Pars ciliaris retinae
8. Elastic fiber	20. Pectinate ligament
9. Filtration angle	21. Posterior chamber
10. Germinal zone	22. Sclera
11. Iris	23. Scleral venous plexus
12. Lens	24. Spaces of Fontana
	25. Vascular layer, choroid

Figure 19.2. Eye, Dog. Anterior, peripheral portion of the eye.

Figure 19.3. Lens, Equator, Horse. Newly formed and older lens fibers are visible in this section through the germinal zone. The latter is the marginal band of lens epithelium that lies around the equator. Its cells are capable of dividing throughout adult life.

Figure 19.4. Ciliary Body, Dog. The epithelium of the ciliary body is called the pars ciliaris retinae. This portion of the nonphotosensitive retina consists of an inner (closer to the cavity of the vitreous humor), nonpigmented layer and an outer, heavily pigmented layer of cells.

Figure 19.5. Ciliary Body, Cat (Orcein). In addition to smooth muscle (see Fig. 19.4), the ciliary body contains an abundance of elastic fibers.

Figure 19.6. Eye, Horse. In a section through a horse's eye, the limbus does not overlap the pectinate ligament. Compare with Figure 19.7. The filtration angle is indicated by the triangular-shaped area marked by the dashed line.

Figure 19.7 ×12.5

Figure 19.8 ×62.5

Figure 19.9 ×62.5

Figure 19.10 ×62.5

Figure 19.11 ×250

KEY	
1. Bulbar conjunctiva	13. Nonpigmented cells
2. Ciliary process	14. Palpebral conjunctiva
3. Cornea	15. Pectinate ligament
4. Corneoscleral trabecular meshwork	16. Pigmented cells
5. Descemet's membrane	17. Pigmented surface cells
6. Filtration angle	18. Sclera
7. Iris	19. Spaces of Fontana
8. Limbus	20. Sphincter muscle
9. Melanocyte	21. Stroma
10. Myoepithelial cell, cytoplasm	22. Uveal trabecular meshwork
11. Myoepithelial cell, nucleus	23. Zonular fibers
12. Myoepithelial cells	

Figure 19.7. Eye, Pig. In a section through the eye of a domestic mammal other than the horse, the limbus overlaps the pectinate ligament. The area of the filtration angle is outlined by dots.

Figure 19.8. Filtration Angle, Pig. Collagenous fibers, elastic fibers, fibroblasts, and pigment cells form the pectinate ligament and the uveal trabecular meshwork. The corneoscleral trabecular meshwork is a three-dimensional latticework of fine fibers of connective tissue and fibroblasts lying adjacent to the sclera.

Figure 19.9. Ciliary Processes, Pig. The nonpigmented cells of the epithelium of the ciliary processes cover the pigmented cells. Together these two layers of cells comprise the pars ciliaris retinae, which extends from the ora ciliaris retinae to the iris. The nonpigmented cells give rise to the zonular fibers.

Figure 19.10. Iris, Horse. The back surface of the iris is covered by a continuation of the pars ciliaris retinae and is called the pars iridica retinae. The surface layer of the pars iridica retinae consists of heavily pigmented cells, and its inner layer is formed by the contractile, pigmented myoepithelial cells that dilate the iris. Anteriorly, the iris is covered by a discontinuous layer of stromal cells.

Figure 19.11. Iris, Dog. The heavily pigmented cells of the pars iridica retinae cover the posterior surface of the iris. The myoepithelial cells of the pars iridica retinae are partially pigmented in the region of their nuclei.

Figure 19.12 ×625

Figure 19.16 ×62.5

Figure 19.13 ×12.5

Figure 19.12. Iris, Cat. In the cat the melanocytes of the iris are binucleate and contain rod-shaped melanosomes.

Figure 19.13. Corpus Nigrum, Goat. In ungulates the pupillary border of the iris is differentiated into corpora nigra, which are vascularized outgrowths of the stroma and pigmented epithelium of the iris.

Figure 19.14. Cornea, Dog. The anterior surface is covered by a nonkeratinized stratified squamous epithelium. The posterior surface is covered by squamous or low cuboidal cells.

Figure 19.15. Junction of Cornea and Bulbar Conjunctiva, Pig. Both the cornea and bulbar conjunctiva are covered by a nonkeratinized stratified squamous epithelium at their junction. The basal border of the conjunctiva is irregular, and the cells of its deepest layers are smaller than those of the anterior epithelium of the cornea.

Figure 19.16. Ora Ciliaris Retinae, Dog. The transition zone between the photosensitive and the nonphotosensitive (pars ciliaris retinae) regions of the retina is named the ora ciliaris retinae.

Figure 19.14 ×62.5

Figure 19.15 ×125

Figure 19.17 ×25

Figure 19.20 ×250

Figure 19.18 ×125

KEY	
1. Blood vessel	13. Nerve fibers, bundle of
2. Choriocapillary layer	14. Optic disc
3. Choroid	15. Optic nerve
4. Cone	16. Outer nuclear layer
5. Ganglion cell layer	17. Outer plexiform layer
6. Inner limiting membrane	18. Pigment epithelium
7. Inner nuclear layer	19. Retina
8. Inner plexiform layer	20. Rod
9. Lamina cribrosa	21. Sclera
10. Layer of rods and cones	22. Tapetum lucidum
11. Melanocytes	23. Vascular layer, choroid
12. Nerve fiber layer	

Figure 19.17. Optic Nerve, sagittal section, Dog. Nerve fibers of the retina converge to form the optic nerve at the optic disc (blind spot).

Figure 19.18. Lamina Cribrosa, x.s., Dog. At the lamina cribrosa the connective tissue of the sclera forms a sievelike framework, which subdivides the optic nerve into bundles of fibers.

Figure 19.19. Retina, Choroid, and Part of the Sclera, Pig. Note that the dendrites (cones) of cone cells of the pig are particularly plump and easily recognized.

Figure 19.20. Fibrous Tapetum Lucidum, Sheep. The tapetum lucidum of ruminants and horses is a compact membrane of connective tissue sandwiched between the choriocapillary and vascular layers of the choroid. The cells of the pigment epithelium of the retina contain few or no pigment granules where a tapetum lucidum is present. Compare with Figure 19.21.

Figure 19.19 ×180

Figure 19.21

×250

Figure 19.25

×12.5

Figure 19.22

×250

KEY	
1. Anterior chamber	13. Melanocytes
2. Bulbar conjunctiva	14. Nerve fiber layer
3. Capillary, x.s.	15. Nictitating membrane, bulbar
4. Choriocapillary layer	surface
5. Cornea	16. Outer nuclear layer
6. Cytoplasmic process	17. Outer plexiform layer
7. Descemet's membrane	18. Pectinate ligament
8. Elastic cartilage	19. Pigment epithelium
9. Ganglion cell layer	20. Sclera
10. Inner nuclear layer	21. Tapetal cell
11. Inner plexiform layer	22. Tapetum lucidum
12. Layer of rods and cones	23. Vascular layer, choroid

Figure 19.21. Retina, Choroid, and Part of the Sclera, Dog. Where the tapetum lucidum is lacking from the choroid layer, the cells of the pigment epithelium of the retina contain numerous melanosomes.

Figure 19.22. Cellular Tapetum Lucidum, Dog. In profile, the cells of the tapetum lucidum of carnivores are bricklike. Note that in this section the cells of the pigment epithelium of the retina are indistinct and lack pigment. Compare with Figure 19.21.

Figure 19.23. Melanocytes of Choroid Layer, Dog. Melanocytes of the choroid layer are flat polygonal cells with cytoplasmic processes. Their polygonal shape is evident in this tangential cut through the choroid layer.

Figure 19.24. Tapetum Lucidum, Dog. Tapetal cells are flattened and have a pentagonal or hexagonal outline, which is apparent in this tangential section through the choroid layer. The cells are filled with numerous small rods, whose long axes parallel the flat surfaces of the cells.

Figure 19.25. Nictitating Membrane and Cornea, Horse. A portion of the bulbar surface of the nictitating membrane and its supportive cartilage are shown. The nictitating membrane is a fold of the ventromedial portion of the conjunctiva. It contains elastic cartilage in the horse, pig, and cat and hyaline cartilage in the dog and ruminants.

Figure 19.23

×250

Figure 19.24

×625

254 COLOR ATLAS OF **VETERINARY HISTOLOGY**

Figure 19.26   ×12.5

Figure 19.27   ×125

Figure 19.28   ×62.5

Figure 19.29   ×12.5

Figure 19.30   ×125

KEY	
1. Diffuse lymphatic tissue	9. Serous acinus
2. Duct	10. Stratified columnar epithelium
3. Epidermis	11. Stratified squamous epithelium
4. Goblet cell	12. Superficial gland
5. Hair follicle	13. Sweat gland
6. Hyaline cartilage	14. Tarsal gland
7. Mucous acinus	15. Tarsus
8. Palpebral conjunctiva	

Figure 19.26. Superficial Gland of the Nictitating Membrane, Dog. The base of the cartilage of the nictitating membrane is surrounded by the superficial gland.

Figure 19.27. Superficial Gland of the Nictitating Membrane, Dog. This gland is mixed in the dog and ruminants. It is serous in the horse and cat and mucous in the pig.

Figure 19.28. Palpebral Conjunctiva, Pig. The palpebral conjunctiva is a mucous membrane that lines the inner surface of the eyelid. Its stratified epithelium varies from squamous through columnar and may even appear transitional. Goblet cells may be present.

Figure 19.29. Eyelid, Lower, Horse. The outer surface of the eyelid is covered by thin skin, while the inner surface is lined by the palpebral conjunctiva. The tarsal gland is a multilobulated gland whose duct opens onto the palpebral surface near the margin of the eyelid. The tarsal gland is surrounded by a condensed layer of connective tissue, the tarsus.

Figure 19.30. Eyelid, Upper, Pig. Numerous tubular sweat glands (and sebaceous glands, not shown) occur in the skin surface of the eyelid of the pig.

Figure 19.31 ×12.5

Figure 19.35 ×125

Figure 19.32 ×62.5

Figure 19.31. Eyelid, Lower, Goat. The skin surface of the eyelid contains hair follicles, sweat glands, and sebaceous glands.

Figure 19.32. Eyelid, Lower, Goat. Bundles of smooth and skeletal muscle fibers are scattered in the connective tissue between the tarsus and the skin surface of the eyelid.

Figure 19.33. Krause's Gland, Pig. Krause's gland is a small, accessory lacrimal gland (serous in this preparation) located near the fornix of the conjunctiva.

Figure 19.34. Harderian Gland, Pig. Among domestic mammals this gland is present only in the pig. It secretes a fatty product.

Figure 19.35. Lacrimal Gland, Cow. A compound tubular acinar gland. The lacrimal gland is predominantly a serous gland in ruminants and horses.

Figure 19.33 ×62.5

Figure 19.34 ×250

Figure 19.36

Figure 19.39   ×62.5

KEY	
1. Annular pad	15. Lens body
2. Anterior chamber	16. Lens fibers, annular pad
3. Brücke's muscle	17. Lens fibers, lens body
4. Bulbar conjunctiva	18. Nonpigmented epithelium, iris
5. Canal of Schlemm	19. Pectinate ligament
6. Capsule	20. Pigmented epithelium, iris
7. Cavity of the lens	21. Posterior chamber
8. Cavity of vitreous	22. Sclera
humor	23. Scleral cartilage
9. Ciliary body	24. Scleral ossicle
10. Ciliary process	25. Scleral trabecular meshwork
11. Cornea	26. Spaces of Fontana
12. Crampton's muscle	27. Sphincter muscle
13. Dilator muscle	28. Zonular fibers
14. Iris	

Figure 19.37   ×125

Figure 19.36. Eye, Drawing of an Anterolateral Segment, Chicken.

Figure 19.37. Lens, Chicken. A portion of the annular pad and lens body.

Figure 19.38. Filtration Angle, Chicken. The filtration angle is bordered by the cornea, iris, ciliary body, and sclera in the chicken. It is bridged by a trabecular meshwork of the pectinate ligament, which encloses the spaces of Fontana.

Figure 19.39. Ciliary Process, Chicken (Masson's). Ciliary processes occur below the base of the iris and fuse with the lens capsule of the annular pad. The ciliary epithelium also attaches to the capsule by zonular fibers.

Figure 19.38   ×25

Figure 19.40

×250

Figure 19.41

×125

Figure 19.42

×250

Figure 19.43

×62.5

Figure 19.44

×62.5

KEY	
1. Bowman's membrane	10. Posterior epithelium
2. Ciliary body	11. Scleral cartilage
3. Descemet's membrane	12. Scleral ossicle
4. Dilator muscle cell	13. Space artifact
5. Elastic fiber	14. Sphincter muscle cell
6. Lipid vacuole	15. Squamous cell, nucleus
7. Nonpigmented epithelium, iris	16. Stratified squamous epithelium
8. Pectinate ligament	17. Stroma
9. Pigmented epithelium, iris	18. Zonular fibers

Figure 19.40. Iris, Chicken. The iridial musculature of the chicken is composed of skeletal muscle cells, which are characterized by the presence of numerous lipid vacuoles. Unlike mammals, the anterior (corneal) surface of the iris is covered by a layer of flattened, nonpigmented epithelial cells. The posterior (lens) surface of the iris (see Fig. 19.39) is covered by a stratified pigmented epithelium that is three to five cells thick.

Figure 19.41. Junction of Ciliary Body and Iris, Chicken (Orcein). The elastic fibers of the pectinate ligament insert into an elastic meshwork of the ciliary body.

Figure 19.42. Pectinate Ligament, Chicken. The elastic fibers of the pectinate ligament are covered by a simple squamous epithelium.

Figure 19.43. Cornea, Chicken. A well.developed Bowman's membrane separates the anterior, stratified squamous epithelium of the cornea from the underlying stroma.

Figure 19.44. Sclera, Chicken. The sclera is strengthened anteriorly by overlapping bony plates (scleral ossicles). Posteriorly, it consists of a thin layer of cartilage. See Figure 19.36 for the location of ossicles and cartilage. The region of overlap of these skeletal elements is shown here. In this section the ciliary body has separated from the sclera, creating a space artifact.

Figure 19.45 ×62.5

Figure 19.46 ×250

Figure 19.47 ×12.5

Figure 19.48 ×250

Figure 19.49 ×125

KEY	
1. Blood vessels	12. Melanocyte
2. Bridge	13. Nerve fiber layer
3. Capillary	14. Optic nerve
4. Choriocapillary layer	15. Outer nuclear layer
5. Choroid	16. Outer plexiform layer
6. Covering membrane	17. Pecten
7. Ganglion cell layer	18. Pigment epithelium
8. Inner nuclear layer	19. Retina
9. Inner plexiform layer	20. Scleral cartilage
10. Layer of rods and cones	21. Space
11. Loose connective tissue	

Figure 19.45. Retina and Choroid, Chicken. The bulk of the choroid is composed of blood vessels and large spaces supported by a loose connective tissue. The layers of the retina are comparable with those of mammals.

Figure 19.46. Retina and Choroid, Chicken. Cells of the pigment epithelium of the retina are tall and contain rod.shaped pigment granules. The basal region of each cell contains the nucleus and a few pigment granules.

Figure 19.47. Pecten, Chicken. The pecten is a thin, folded, and heavily pigmented membrane that projects into the vitreous humor from the posteroventral surface of the eye.

Figure 19.48. Pecten, Chicken. Numerous, polymorphic melanocytes are interspersed through this highly vascularized, nutritive membrane. The large capillaries are lined by thick endothelial cells with plump nuclei.

Figure 19.49. Bridge of Pecten, Chicken. This thickened, highly pigmented mass of pectineal tissue is located along the free edge of the pecten.

Figure 19.50

×62.5

Figure 19.50. Eyelid, Chicken. A thin epidermis covers the eyelid. Herbst corpuscles are associated with a feather follicle.

Figure 19.51. Lacrimal Gland, Chicken. This compound tubular gland produces a mucoid secretion and is organized into lobules.

Figure 19.52. Harderian Gland, Chicken. This accessory immunologic gland contains a multitude of plasma cells. It is located on the dorsal posterior surface of the eye.

Figure 19.53. Harderian Gland, Chicken. Detail of the Harderian gland showing numerous plasma cells surrounding the vacuolated cells of the tubular secretory units.

Figure 19.51

×25

Figure 19.52

×25

Figure 19.53

×250

20

THE EAR

Sensations of sound and balance are received by separate and specialized areas of the ear before being transmitted to the brain, where they are interpreted. Based on anatomy, location, and function, the ear is divisible into external, middle, and internal components. The **external ear** collects sound waves, which it channels to the tympanic membrane. Vibrations produced in the latter are transmitted by the ossicles of the **middle ear** to fluids of the **internal ear,** where they generate movements of the delicate basilar membrane. Such movements stimulate sensory hair cells from which impulses are relayed by sensory nerves to the brain, where the sound is identified.

MAMMALS

The external ear of domestic mammals is comprised of the **pinna** (auricle), which collects sound, and an **external auditory meatus,** which conveys the sound waves to the **tympanic membrane.**

The external auditory meatus is lined by a continuation of the surface skin. Hair, sebaceous glands, and tubular ceruminous glands are present. The combined secretions of these glands, plus sloughed epithelial cells, form cerumen (ear wax). The outer portion of the meatus is supported by cartilage, the remainder by bone.

Middle-ear ossicles (**malleus, incus,** and **stapes**) are located in the **tympanic cavity.** They bridge the cavity from the tympanic membrane to the oval window located within the petrous part of the temporal bone.

The tympanic cavity is surrounded by bone. The tympanic membrane forms the lateral wall of the cavity. It is composed of a thin, outer layer of epithelium that is continuous with the skin of the external auditory meatus; a thin layer of connective tissue; and an inner layer of simple squamous or cuboidal epithelium. The remainder of the cavity is lined by ciliated columnar and simple squamous cells. The latter cover the ossicles, as well as portions of the wall of the cavity.

The **membranous labyrinth** of the inner ear consists of the **cochlear duct, sacculus, utriculus,** and **semicircular ducts.** Cavities within the petrous segment of the temporal bone, lined by periosteum and containing **perilymph** (a fluid similar to cerebrospinal fluid), house the membranous labyrinth. Those cavities containing the semicircular ducts are called the **semicircular canals;** the one containing the sacculus and utriculus is called the **vestibule;** and the one containing the **cochlear duct** (membranous cochlea, scala media) is named the **cochlear canal** (bony cochlea). The cochlear canal spirals like a snail shell around a central pillar of bone, the **modiolus.** A thin shelf of bone, the **osseous spiral lamina,** travels up the modiolus like the thread of a screw. The number of turns in the cochlear canal varies. There are two and one-half in the horse, three in the cat, and four in the pig, for example.

Each semicircular duct is lined by a mesothelium, is filled with **endolymph,** and bears an expansion, the **ampulla.** A sensory structure, the **crista ampullaris,** is located in each ampulla. The **sensory hair cells** and **supporting cells** of each crista are covered by a **gelatinous cupula.** When the latter is deflected during rotational movements of the head, the sensory cells are stimulated and impulses are sent to the brain, where the signals are interpreted.

Both the sacculus and utriculus are filled with endolymph and are lined, in part, by **maculae,** which are patchlike collections of sensory hair cells and supporting cells. The remainder of these structures is lined by mesothelium. Embedded in the outer surface of the gelatinous otolithic membrane covering the maculae are numerous crystalline particles of calcium carbonate called **otoliths** (otoconia, statoconia). As the membrane shifts in response to gravity acting on the otoliths, sensory cells of the maculae are stimulated. Impulses sent to the brain in response to the stimulus make the animal aware of the position of its head in space. Also, because of the effect of inertia on the otolithic membranes when the body suddenly begins to move or slow down, hair cells are stimulated and the sensations of acceleration and deceleration are experienced.

The spirally organized cochlear duct is filled with endolymph and is roughly triangular in cross section. One side of the duct is attached to the **spiral ligament,** a thickening of the periosteal lining of the cochlear canal. This side consists of a stratified cuboidal epithelium, the **stria vascularis.** Capillaries occur among the superficial cuboidal cells of the stria. The side of the duct opposite the stria is pointed. The floor of the duct is formed from the fibrous **basilar membrane,** which extends from the spiral ligament to the osseous spiral lamina. The roof is formed from the **vestibular (Reissner's) membrane,** which consists of two adjacent layers of simple squamous epithelium. Above the roof is a large chamber, the **scala vestibuli,** which is filled with perilymph. Below the floor of the cochlear duct is another large chamber filled with perilymph, the **scala tympani.** All three scalas follow a spiral path to the top of the cochlear canal. At the apex the scala vestibuli communicates with the scala tympani through a tiny opening called the **helicotrema.**

The upper surface of the basilar membrane supports the acoustically sensitive **organ of Corti,** which is bathed by the endolymph within the cochlear duct. The lower surface of the basilar membrane is lined by a simple squamous epithelium that faces the scala tympani. The organ of Corti is comprised of sensory hair cells and various different supporting cells. Overlying the organ of Corti and extending from the **spiral limbus** (an elevation of connective tissue above the osseous spiral lamina) is the proteinaceous, **tectorial membrane.** Stereocilia of the sensory cells of the organ of Corti contact the tectorial membrane. The stereocilia are displaced when the basilar membrane vibrates in response to sound waves passing through the fluid-filled scalas. The sensory cells respond to this perturbation by initiating impulses in the cochlear nerve, which are transmitted to the brain for interpretation. The stimulatory sound waves are dissipated through the secondary tympanic membrane of the round window located in the lower part of the medial wall of the tympanic cavity.

CHICKEN

The ear of the chicken consists of the same basic components as that of the mammal, but there are some differences.

Although an external auditory meatus is present in the chicken, it is relatively short, and there is no pinna.

The middle ear is lined by a cuboidal epithelium that also covers the columella, a single partially ossified rod that extends from the tympanic membrane to the oval window. The **columella** transmits vibrations from the tympanic membrane to the internal ear, taking the place of the malleus, incus, and stapes of mammals.

Unlike mammals, the sacculus of the internal ear contains two maculae. The cochlear duct is a short, narrow, slightly curved tube. It possesses a terminal expansion, the **lagena,** a structure peculiar to birds. The lagena contains a macula that is similar in structure and function to other maculae (see under Mammals). The cochlear duct is separated from the overlying scala vestibuli by the **tegmentum vasculosum.** The latter is composed of a thin membrane of connective tissue integrated with a highly folded epithelium containing numerous blood vessels. The epithelium faces the cavity of the cochlear duct. The tegmentum occupies the same position as the vestibular membrane in mammals. The common wall separating the cochlear duct from the scala tympani below is formed from the basilar membrane, a platform that supports the organ of Corti (papilla acustica or basilaris). As in mammals, the organ of Corti is composed of sensory and supporting cells and is overlain by a tectorial membrane that is in contact with the sensory hairs (stereocilia) of the sensory cells.

Figure 20.1 ×25

Figure 20.2 ×25

Figure 20.3 ×25

Figure 20.4 ×250

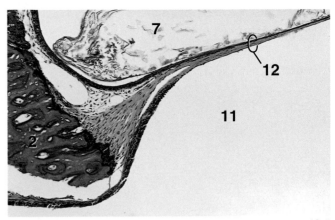

Figure 20.5 ×62.5

KEY		
1. Adipose tissue		7. External auditory meatus
2. Bone		8. Hair follicle
3. Ceruminous gland		9. Pigment granules
4. Duct		10. Sebaceous gland
5. Elastic cartilage		11. Tympanic cavity
6. Epidermis		12. Tympanic membrane

Figure 20.1. External Auditory Meatus, Puppy. The outer portion of the meatus is supported by elastic cartilage. The thin epidermis is underlain by numerous sebaceous glands and a few ceruminous glands. Small hair follicles are present.

Figure 20.2. External Auditory Meatus, Puppy. The external auditory meatus, near the tympanic membrane, contains large sebaceous glands.

Figure 20.3. External Auditory Meatus, Goat. Outer portion of the meatus with numerous ceruminous glands. Hair follicles and portions of sebaceous glands are also present.

Figure 20.4. Ceruminous Gland, Goat. The secretory epithelium of these apocrine glands varies from cuboidal to columnar. The cells contain tiny, brown pigment granules.

Figure 20.5. Tympanic Membrane, Periphery, Puppy. The tympanic membrane has a core of collagenous fibers. Its outer (external auditory meatus) surface is covered by a stratified squamous epithelium; its inner (tympanic cavity) surface is covered by a simple squamous or cuboidal epithelium.

Figure 20.6 ×12.5

Figure 20.10 ×125

Figure 20.7 ×250

Figure 20.8 ×12.5

Figure 20.6. Malleus and Tympanic Membrane, Puppy. The handle (manubrium) of the malleus is attached to the tympanic membrane.

Figure 20.7. Tympanic Membrane, Puppy. Where the manubrium of the malleus is embedded in the tympanic membrane, the connective tissue of the tympanic membrane is thicker than elsewhere, and blood vessels are abundant.

Figure 20.8. Portion of Stapes and Incus, Puppy. The footplate of the stapes is attached to the oval window by an annular ligament (broken on one side in this section). The stapes articulates with the lenticular process of the incus.

Figure 20.9. Joint, Malleus and Incus, Puppy. The head of the malleus articulates with the body of the incus in this synovial joint.

Figure 20.10. Junction of Lenticular Process and Stapes, Puppy. The stapes articulates with the lenticular process of the incus. See Figure 20.8 for orientation.

Figure 20.9 ×25

Figure 20.11

×125

KEY
1. Ampulla, cavity   8. Pseudostratified epithelium
2. Annular ligament   9. Sensory cell, nucleus
3. Connective tissue   10. Stapes, articular cartilage
4. Cupula, portion of   11. Supporting cell, nucleus
5. Mixed glands   12. Temporal bone, petrous part
6. Otolith   13. Type 1 cell
7. Otolithic membrane

Figure 20.11. Annular Ligament, Stapes, Puppy. The stapes is fastened to the circular cartilage of the oval window by the fibroelastic, annular ligament. See Figure 20.8 for orientation.

Figure 20.12. Macula of Sacculus, Puppy. Otoliths are embedded in a gelatinous otolithic membrane, which lies on an epithelium consisting of sensory and supporting cells. Chalicelike, Type I sensory cells and the basal nuclei of supporting cells are evident in this micrograph.

Figure 20.13. Crista Ampullaris, Puppy. This ridge of sensory epithelium, supported by connective tissue, protrudes into the ampulla of a semicircular duct and is oriented at right angles to the long axis of the duct. The epithelium consists of sensory and supporting cells similar to those found in the maculae. A mass of gelatinous material, the cupula, covers the surface epithelium.

Figure 20.14. Guttural Pouch, Horse. This diverticulum of the eustachian tube is lined by a ciliated, pseudostratified columnar epithelium with goblet cells. Mixed glands occur in the lamina propria.

Figure 20.12

×250

Figure 20.13

×125

Figure 20.14

×62.5

Figure 20.15   ×18

Figure 20.16   ×90

KEY	
1. Basilar membrane	10. Spiral ganglion
2. Cochlear duct	11. Spiral ligament
3. Cochlear nerve	12. Spiral limbus
4. Inner tunnel	13. Spiral tunnel
5. Modiolus	14. Stria vascularis
6. Organ of Corti	15. Tectorial membrane
7. Osseous spiral lamina	16. Temporal bone, petrous part
8. Scala tympani	17. Vestibular membrane
9. Scala vestibuli	

Figure 20.15. Cochlea, Puppy. Cross section through a portion of the spiral cochlea. See Figure 20.16 for details of cochlear duct region.

Figure 20.16. Cochlea, Puppy. Detail of the region of the cochlear duct (scala media, membranous cochlea).

Figure 20.17

×62.5

Figure 20.17. Semicircular Canal, x.s., Chicken. The semicircular canal is a part of the bony labyrinth. It contains the semicircular duct, a part of the membranous labyrinth. The duct is lined by a simple squamous epithelium except at the raphe, where cuboidal cells form the lining.

Figure 20.18. Cochlea, x.s., Chicken (Masson's).

Figure 20.19. Organ of Corti, Cochlea, x.s., Chicken (Masson's).

Figure 20.20. Tegmentum Vasculosum, Cochlea, Chicken (Masson's). This thick membrane rests on a thin base of connective tissue and possesses a highly folded epithelial surface with numerous vascular loops. The epithelium consists of light and dark cells. Dark cells have a constricted neck region that extends to the surface of the epithelium. Their basal portion contains the nucleus and is irregularly shaped. The cytoplasm is very dense. Light cells have a pale cytoplasm and surround the dark cells.

Figure 20.18

×62.5

Figure 20.19

×250

Figure 20.20

×250

GLOSSARY

A band: The part of a sarcomere, of both skeletal and cardiac muscle cells, containing actin and myosin myofilaments and located centrally between the I bands of the sarcomere.

Abomasum: The glandular stomach of a ruminant.

Accessory gland: The name applied to any of the following glands of the male reproductive system: bulbourethral, prostate, seminal vesicle.

Acid stain (anionic stain): A dye, used for histologic or cytologic staining procedures, that carries a negative charge. Such dyes attach electrostatically to positively charged components of cells or other tissue elements.

Acidophil (alpha cell): An acidophilic chromophil found within the pars distalis of the pituitary.

Acidophilic: A cell or tissue component that is selectively stained by an acid dye.

Acinus: A small grape-shaped secretory unit of an acinar gland or tubuloacinar gland.

Adenohypophysis: The glandular portion of the pituitary. It is derived during development from Rathke's pouch. It includes the pars distalis, pars tuberalis, and the pars intermedia.

Adipocyte: Synonym for fat cell.

Adipose tissue: Aggregates of adipocytes within loose connective tissue.

Adrenal cortex: That part of the adrenal gland surrounding the medulla. It is divisible into four zones of cells that produce steroid hormones.

Adrenal medulla: The region interior to the cortex of the adrenal gland. The chromaffin cells of the medulla secrete the hormones epinephrine (adrenalin) and norepinephrine.

Adventitia: The external layer of connective tissue covering a structure.

Afferent arteriole: Smallest branch of the renal artery that delivers blood directly to the glomerulus of a renal corpuscle.

Agranulocyte: A leukocyte that lacks specific granules, e.g., a lymphocyte or monocyte.

Air capillary: In birds, a tiny respiratory tubule forming part of a network connecting parabronchi. Respiratory exchange occurs between the blood in surrounding blood capillaries and the gas within air capillaries.

Air sac: One of several rather large, thin-walled, and air-filled sacs found within various parts of the body cavity of a bird. Many hollow bones of the chicken contain extensions of air sacs. The designation air sac is also used as a synonym for alveolus.

Alveolar bone: The bone lining the alveolus (root socket) of a tooth. Collagenous fibers attach the root of the tooth to the alveolar bone.

Alveolar duct: The portion of the respiratory tree of a mammal lying between a respiratory duct and an alveolar sac.

Alveolar sac: A terminal, baglike expansion of the bronchial tree whose wall is formed entirely from alveoli.

Alveolar septum: All of the tissue separating the cavities of adjacent alveoli of the lung.

Alveolus: One of millions of thin-walled, tiny sacs forming the terminal limits of the bronchial tree. It is sometimes called an air sac. The term is also used as a synonym for the acinus of a exocrine gland.

Ameloblasts: Cells that form the enamel organ of a tooth and produce the enamel.

Amorphous ground substance: A viscous and colorless material that fills the spaces between the fibers, cells, and vessels of connective tissue.

Ampulla: A dilated portion of a tubular structure such as the ampulla of a semicircular duct of the inner ear, or the ampulla of the vas deferens.

Anal gland: A tubuloacinar gland found within the submucosa and muscularis of the anal canal of carnivores and pigs.

Anal sac: One of a pair of pouchlike glands found within the tissue adjacent to the anus.

Anastomosis: A connection between two structures.

Anestrus: In nonprimate mammals, the period of sexual inactivity.

Annular ligament: A fibroelastic ligament that attaches the stapes of the middle ear to the cartilage of the oval window.

Annular pad: The portion of the lens of the chicken eye located around the equator of the lens.

Annular sinus: A large blood sinus lying between the inner and outer layers of the connective tissue sheath of a sinus hair follicle.

Anterior chamber: The space, filled with aqueous humor, that is bounded by the cornea, iris, and lens of the eye.

Anterior epithelium: The stratified squamous epithelium of the outer surface of the cornea.

Antrum: A cavity such as the antrum of an ovarian follicle.

Aortic body: A small encapsulated structure, located between the pulmonary artery and aorta, that contains blood vessels, nerves, and two kinds of parenchyma cells.

Apocrine gland: A gland whose secretory cells release their product by pinching off blebs of cytoplasm containing secretory product from their free surface.

Arachnoid layer: The middle meninx enveloping the spinal cord and brain.

Argyrophilic: A substance having an affinity for silver.

Arrector pili muscle: The smooth muscle originating from the dermis of the skin and inserting on the connective tissue sheath of a hair follicle. Elevates the hair.

Arteriole: The smallest of the arteries. Consists of an endothelium and one or two layers of smooth muscle.

Arteriovenous shunt: A vessel that enables blood to flow directly from an artery to a vein without passing through a capillary bed.

Artery: A blood vessel that carries blood away from the heart to a capillary bed.

Artifact: Any alteration in appearance or structure that has been caused by artificial means.

Arytenoid cartilage: One of two small cartilages located at the back of the larynx.

Astrocyte: A neuroglial cell having long processes and a starlike appearance.

Atresia: The degenerative regression of an ovarian follicle.

Atretic follicle: An ovarian follicle that has undergone atresia.

Atrium: A cavity or chamber such as an atrium of the heart or an air vesicle of a chicken's parabronchus.

Auerbach's plexus: A collection of nerve cells and fibers lying between the circular and longitudinal layers of the muscularis externa of the digestive tract.

Axon hillock: The place of origin of an axon from a nerve cell body. The hillock lacks Nissl granules.

Azurophilic granule: Nonspecific granules found in the cytoplasm of some leukocytes.

Band cell: A granulocyte in the process of development and characterized by the presence of a straplike unsegmented nucleus.

Barb: A subdivision, bearing barbules, of a vane of a contour feather. The barbules of adjacent barbs interlock with one another by means of their hooklets.

Barb stem: The stalk of the barb of a feather.

Barbule: A projection, bearing hooklets, from a barb.

Basal cell: A pale cell found in the fundus of the gastric glands of the ventriculus of the chicken. The term basal cell is also applied to a cell attached to the basement membrane of a stratified epithelium.

Basement membrane: A fibrous membrane separating the cells of an epithelium from the underlying connective tissue.

Basic stain (cationic stain): A dye used for histologic or cytologic staining procedures that carries a positive charge. Such stains attach electrostatically to negatively charged elements within cells and tissues.

Basilar membrane: A membrane of the inner ear that supports the organ of Corti.

Basophil: A granulocyte characterized by large, basophilic, specific granules. Also, a cell of the pars distalis of the pituitary gland.

Basophilic: A cell or tissue component that attracts and becomes colored by a basic stain.

Basophilic erythroblast: A developing cell of the erythroid line characterized by an intensely basophilic cytoplasm and a large, round, and deeply stained nucleus.

Bile canaliculus: A tiny channel, formed from the cell membranes of adjacent hepatocytes, that receives bile from the hepatocyte and delivers it to a bile ductule.

Bile ductule: A subdivision of a bile duct found within a portal area (tract) and lined by a simple cuboidal epithelium.

Bistratified epithelium: A stratified epithelium consisting of two layers of cells.

Blastocyst: The vesicular embryonic stage of a mammal that consists of an inner cell mass and outer cell mass (trophoblast) surrounding a fluid-filled cavity (blastocele, blastocyst cavity).

Bone marrow (active): The site of the formation of blood cells (hematopoiesis) within the marrow cavity of a bone.

Bone matrix: The hard, calcified substance of a bone, consisting of hydroxyapatites and collagenous fibers.

Bowman's capsule: The hollow, bulbus, initial portion of a renal corpuscle. Its outer wall is the capsular epithelium (simple squamous), and its inner wall or glomerular epithelium is composed of podocytes.

Bowman's gland: A mucoserous gland located in the lamina propria below the respiratory epithelium. Its duct opens onto the respiratory epithelium.

Bowman's membrane: A membrane of connective tissue that lies below the anterior epithelium of the cornea.

Brain sand: A granular, calcified material that may be found in various parts of the brain.

Bronchiole: A subdivision of the bronchial tree that begins at the termination of the smallest bronchus. Bronchioles vary in diameter, amount of smooth muscle present, and whether a ciliated epithelium is present.

Bronchus: Any subdivision of the bronchial tree from the end of the trachea to a bronchiole. All bronchi are supported by cartilage and are lined by an epithelium that varies from ciliated pseudostratified columnar in the larger bronchi to ciliated simple columnar in the smaller ones.

Bruch's membrane: A thin, refractile membrane of the retina separating the choriocapillary layer of the choroid from the pigment epithelium of the retina.

Brücke's muscle: A ciliary muscle (skeletal) of the chicken eye.

Brunner's gland (duodenal or submucosal gland): A compound tubuloacinar mucous gland found within the submucosa, and to some degree the lamina propria, of the duodenum.

Brush border: A border formed from numerous microvilli of variable length on the apical surface of certain epithelial cells, e.g., those of the proximal convoluted tubules of the kidney.

Buffy coat: The thin layer of leukocytes between the plasma and packed red blood cells in a sample of blood that has been centrifuged.

Bulbar conjunctiva: That portion of the conjunctiva located on the surface of the eyeball.

Bulbourethral gland (Cowper's gland): An accessory male reproductive gland that empties into the urethra. Its secretion forms part of the seminal fluid.

Bursa of Fabricius: A saclike lymphatic diverticulum from the dorsal surface of the proctodeum of birds.

Calamus: The hollow quill of a feather.

Calcified cartilage: Cartilage matrix that has become impregnated with calcium salts, as in the zone of calcification of the epiphyseal disc.

Canal of Hering: A tiny channel, lined by simple cuboidal epithelium, that connects a bile canaliculus to a bile ductule within a portal tract (area).

Canal of Schlemm: A channel within the sclera that drains excess aqueous humor from the eye to the circulatory system.

Canaliculi: In bone, tiny channels that contain the processes of osteocytes.

Capillary: A blood vessel ranging from 4 to 12 micrometers in diameter that is networked with other capillaries and located between an arteriole and venule.

Capsular epithelium: The outer simple squamous epithelium of Bowman's capsule.

Capsule of Glisson: A thin layer of connective tissue enveloping the liver.

Cardiac gland: A mucous gland located in the cardiac gland region of the glandular stomach.

Cardiac gland region: The proximal part of the glandular stomach preceding the fundic gland region.

Cardiac muscle: The striated, involuntary muscle of the heart.

Cardiac skeleton: A supportive framework of connective tissue found at various locations within the wall of the heart.

Caruncle: In ruminants, any nonglandular region of the mucosa of the uterus.

Cavernous space: A thin-walled vein that forms part of the erectile tissue of the urethra.

Cavity of the vitreous humor: A large space behind the lens of the eye that contains a transparent and colorless gelatinous mass, the vitreous body (humor).

Cecum: In mammals, that portion of the large intestine that unites with the small intestine. In chickens, one of two diverticuli that arise from the region of junction of the ileum and large intestine.

Cellular tapetum lucidum: A cellular reflective layer of the choroid of the eye of cats and dogs.

Cementoid (precementum): Uncalcified cementum of a tooth, produced by cells called cementoblasts.

Cementum: A layer of bonelike mineralized tissue covering the dentin of the root of a tooth.

Central artery: A branch of the splenic artery that passes through the white pulp of the spleen.

Central canal: The fluid-filled cavity within the center of the spinal cord.

Central pallor: The pale central area, evident in a surface view, of the biconcave erythrocyte.

Centroacinar cell: An extension of an intercalated duct of the pancreas into the interior of a secretory acinus.

Cerebellum: A part of the brain that lies above the medulla and pons and below the posterior part of the cerebrum.

Cerebrospinal fluid: The clear fluid found within the ventricles of the brain and the central canal of the spinal cord.

Cerumen: A soft, waxy substance formed from the combined secretions of the ceruminous and sebaceous glands of the external auditory meatus and containing sloughed epithelial cells.

Ceruminous gland: A gland of the external auditory meatus whose secretions contribute to the composition of the cerumen.

Cervical os: The opening of the cervix into the vagina.

Chestnut: A small round or oval thickening of the epidermis located on the inner side of the legs of a horse.

Chief cell (stomach): A cell found in the fundic gland region of the stomach that secretes pepsinogen.

Chondrocyte: A cartilage cell surrounded by cartilage matrix.

Chorioallantoic membrane: An extraembryonic membrane of amniotes formed from the fusion of the chorion and the allantois.

Choriocapillary layer: A network of capillaries of the choroid, distributed in a single plane, below Bruch's membrane of the eye.

Chorion laeve: A part of the chorionic sac, having a smooth surface, that is not involved in the formation of the placenta.

Choroid: The portion of the uvea (vascular tunic) of the eye located between the sclera and the photosensitive retina.

Choroid plexus: A highly vascularized portion of the roof of the fourth ventricle and of other ventricles of the brain whose villi are surrounded by cerebrospinal fluid.

Chromaffin cells: Cells of the adrenal medulla that form clusters and anastomosing cords separated by sinusoids.

Chromophil: A cell of the pars distalis of the pituitary that can be stained with various kinds of histologic dye substances.

Chromophobe: A small cell of the pars distalis of the pituitary that stains poorly or not at all with dyes.

Ciliary body: The portion of the uvea between the choroid and the iris.

Ciliary muscle: The musculature of the ciliary body.

Ciliary process: A projection from the surface of the pars ciliaris retinae of the ciliary body to which zonular fibers are attached.

Circumanal gland: A partly sebaceous gland found in the subcutis near the anus of the dog.

Circumferential lamellae: The bony lamellae that lie parallel to the outer and inner surfaces of long bones.

Circumvallate papilla: A large, round elevation bearing numerous taste buds, found on the surface of the tongue.

Classic liver lobule: A cylindrical subunit (about 1 x 2 mm) of the liver that is composed of plates of hepatocytes separated by an extensive network of sinusoids.

Claw: A keratinized derivative of the skin found on the tips of the digits.

Clear cell: A cell of the secretory units of the carpal gland of the pig.

Clearing: In a tissue sample being processed, the replacement of alcohol with a substance miscible with paraffin prior to infiltrating the sample with paraffin.

Clitoris: A structure of the female that is homologous to the glans penis of the male.

Cloaca: A chamber, internal to the vent, of various vertebrates that receives digestive wastes, reproductive cells, and urinary products.

Cochlear canal: The bony canal, within the petrous portion of the temporal bone, that contains the scala tympani, scala media (cochlear duct), and scala vestibuli.

Cochlear duct: A spirally arranged part of the membranous labyrinth, whose walls are formed from the basilar membrane, stria vascularis, and the vestibular membrane.

Collagen: A form of fibrous protein of which several types exist.

Collagenous fibers: Fibers formed from one of the types of the fibrous protein collagen.

Collecting tubule: The part of a uriniferous tubule that receives urine filtrate from a nephron.

Colloid: A gelatinous material found within follicles of the thyroid gland and the pars intermedia of the pituitary gland, among other places.

Columella: An ossicle of the middle ear of birds and some other vertebrates.

Comb: A highly vascularized derivative of the skin found atop the head of the chicken.

Compact bone: A bone whose dense matrix contains few marrow spaces.

Compound follicle: A hair follicle bearing several hair bulbs.

Conjunctiva: An epithelial layer covering part of the bulbar surface of the eye and the inner surface of the eyelid.

Connecting duct: Tubules of the epididymis of the rooster, which are also called excretory canals.

Connective tissue proper: A category of connective tissue that includes loose, dense, reticular, elastic, and adipose tissues.

Connective tissue sheath (of hair follicle): A layer of connective tissue surrounding a hair follicle.

Contour feather: A flight feather of birds with a central shaft consisting of a rachis supporting the vanes and a hollow quill.

Coprodeum: The portion of the cloaca that joins the large intestine.

Cornea: The anterior, transparent portion of the fibrous tunic of the eye.

Corneal stroma (substantia propria): Lamellae of collagenous fibers oriented parallel to the corneal surface and located between Bowman's and Descemet's membranes of the cornea.

Corneoscleral trabecular meshwork: A meshwork of trabeculae of connective tissue, fibroblasts, and pigment cells found in the filtration angle of the eye immediately adjacent of the sclera.

Corneous cells: Keratinized cells of a feather follicle or surface epidermis.

Corneous connection: A strand of tissue extending from the corneous layer of a feather follicle to the calamus of a developing feather.

Corona (of lymphatic nodule): The external layer, consisting of numerous small lymphocytes, of an activated lymphatic nodule.

Corona radiata: The columnar cells abutting the zona pellucida and forming the innermost layer of the cumulus oophorus of an ovarian follicle.

Coronary region: The proximal, peripheral part of the horse's hoof located above the laminae.

Corpora amylacea: Concretions of casein and cellular debris found within the cavities of the secretory units of the mammary gland.

Corpora nigra: Highly vascularized proliferations of the pupillary margin of the iris.

Corpus albicans: Scar tissue remaining following regression of the corpus luteum of the ovary.

Corpus cavernosum: A mass of erectile tissue located within the body of the penis.

Corpus cavernosum clitoridis: Erectile tissue of the clitoris.

Corpus luteum: An endocrine gland derived from granulosa cells and theca interna cells of a postovulatory ovarian follicle; its cells secrete progesterone and estrogen.

Corpus spongiosum (corpus cavernosum urethra): Erectile tissue within the glans of the penis and surrounding the penile urethra.

Cortex (hair): That portion of a hair located between the cuticle and the medulla.

Cortical nephron (chicken): A nephron with a relatively small renal corpuscle located in the cortex of the kidney.

Cotyledonary placenta: The type of placenta found in ruminants where numerous, bean-shaped portions of the chorioallantoic membrane form the functional connections with the endometrium.

Crampton's muscle: One of the ciliary muscles (skeletal) of the chicken's eye.

Crenated: Having a corrugated or scalloped border, e.g., the cell membrane of an erythrocyte following the loss of water.

Crista ampullaris: A sensory structure located within the ampulla of a semicircular duct of the inner ear.

Crop: A caudal diverticulum of the esophagus of the chicken used for the temporary storage of food.

Crypt of Lieberkühn (intestinal gland): A simple tubular gland located within the lamina propria of the small and large intestine.

Cumulus oophorus: The mound of granulosa cells surrounding an oocyte of the ovarian follicle of a mammal.

Cupula: The gelatinous covering of the sensory hair cells of the crista ampullaris.

Cuticle (hair): The layer of flat cells, arranged in a shingle-like manner, on the surface of a hair.

Cytoplasmic bridge: The region of adhesion (at the desmosomes) between adjacent epithelial cells of the stratum spinosum of the epidermis.

Cytotrophoblast: The cellular layer of the trophoblast (covering layer of the blastocyst) that contributes to the formation of the placenta.

Dark zone (glandular stomach): The distal and longest part of the fundic gland region of the stomach of carnivores; characterized by a thick mucosa and relatively shallow gastric pits.

Deciduate placenta: A type of placenta wherein the chorioallantoic membrane has fused with the endometrium.

Dendrite: The neuronal process that receives stimuli.

Dense irregular connective tissue: A form of connective tissue proper that consists of relatively thick collagenous fibers arranged as a feltwork with scant space between them. The predominant cell is the fibroblast.

Dense regular connective tissue: A form of connective tissue proper that consists of relatively thick collagenous fibers, arranged in parallel, with scant space between them. The fibroblast is the only cell type present.

Dental lamina: A band of ectodermal cells from the embryonic jaw that grow into the underlying mesenchyme. Buds from the dental lamina give rise to the primordia of the enamel organs of the teeth.

Dental papilla: A projection of mesenchyme of the embryonic jaw into the developing enamel organ.

Dental pulp: The soft tissue of the pulp cavity of a tooth.

Dental sac: The mesenchymal precursor of the connective tissue surrounding a developing tooth, or the connective tissue surrounding a developing tooth.

Dentin: The ivory that forms the mass of the tooth.

Dermal papilla: A projection of the dermis into the overlying epidermis.

Dermis: The connective tissue of the skin located beneath the epidermis.

Descemet's membrane: An acellular layer separating the stroma from the posterior epithelium of the cornea.

Diaphysis: The shaft of a long bone.

Diencephalon: A subdivision of the brain composed of the thalamus, subthalamus, and hypothalamus.

Diestrus: That part of the estrous cycle, between metestrus and anestrus, when development and secretory activity of the endometrial glands peak.

Diffuse lymphatic tissue: A type of lymphatic tissue characterized by a moderate amount of scattered lymphocytes.

Diffuse placenta: The name given to a placenta when the chorioallantoic membrane makes a major structural contribution.

Digital cushion: The loose connective tissue (subcutis) below the dermis of the digital pad.

Digital pad: The soft, shock-absorbing tissue formed by the epidermis, dermis, and subcutis beneath the digits of many mammals.

Diplokaryocyte: A binucleate giant cell of the epithelium of a chorionic villus of the placenta of the cow.

Distal convoluted tubule: That portion of a nephron located between the loop of Henle and a collecting tubule.

Dorsal plate (claw): The keratinized, upper part of a claw.

Dorsal root ganglion: The ganglion of the dorsal root of a spinal nerve.

Down feather: A soft, fluffy feather that lacks barbules with hooklets.

Duct of the epididymis: The highly convoluted duct forming a major part of the epididymis.

Dura mater: The outer meninx of dense connective tissue surrounding the brain and spinal cord.

Efferent arteriole: The arteriole carrying blood away from the glomerulus of a renal corpuscle.

Efferent ductule: One of several small tubes connecting the rete testis to the duct of the epididymis.

Elastic cartilage: A type of cartilage whose matrix contains numerous elastic fibers.

Elastic fiber: A component of certain connective tissues that forms from the protein elastin.

Ellipsoid: A fusiform structure, composed of macrophages, that surrounds a portion of each of the capillaries of the penicillus of the spleen.

Embedding: When an infiltrated tissue is transferred to a fresh solution of embedding medium (e.g. melted paraffin) and the paraffin is then allowed to harden.

Embryonal connective tissue: A form of connective tissue exemplified by mesenchyme and mucous connective tissue.

Enamel: The hard, glistening material covering the exposed surface of a tooth.

Endocardium: The tissue layer lining the atria and ventricles of the heart.

Endochondral bone: Bone that has been formed by replacing a cartilaginous model.

Endocrine gland: A ductless gland.

Endolymph: A clear fluid contained within the semicircular ducts, sacculus, utriculus, and cochlear duct of the inner ear.

Endometrial gland: A simple tubular gland of the endometrium of the uterus.

Endometrium: The mucosa of the uterus.

Endomysium: The connective tissue immediately surrounding individual muscle cells of a fascicle of a muscle.

Endoneurium: The connective tissue immediately surrounding the processes of nerve cells within a fascicle of a nerve.

Endosteum: The layer of squamous osteogenic cells lining the entire marrow cavity and extending into the haversian canals.

Endotheliochorial placenta: A type of placenta, found in carnivores, where the maternal and fetal blood are separated by four layers of tissue.

Endothelium: The simple squamous epithelium lining the cardiovascular system and lymphatic vessels.

Enterochromaffin cell: A form of APUD cell (amine-precursor uptake decarboxylase cell) found in the gastrointestinal tract, among other places; it can be stained with bichromate solutions and produces either a hormone or a paracrine (a substance that acts locally by diffusing to a target organ).

Eosinophil: A granulocyte characterized by the presence of eosinophilic specific granules.

Ependymal cell: A neuroglial cell that lines the ventricles of the brain and the central canal of the spinal cord.

Epicardium: The outermost layer of the heart.

Epidermal collar: A thick ring of epidermal cells situated at the base of the follicle of a feather.

Epidermal laminae: The platelike epidermal structures of the wall of the horse's hoof.

Epidermal peg: A downward extension of the epidermis that alternates with upward-extending dermal papillae.

Epidermis: The ectodermally derived stratified squamous epithelium forming the surface layer of the skin.

Epididymis: A highly coiled tube of the male reproductive system located between the efferent ductules and the vas deferens.

Epimysium: The outer sheath of connective tissue of a muscle.

Epineurium: The outer sheath of connective tissue of a nerve.

Epiphyseal disc: A plate of hyaline cartilage between the epiphysis and diaphysis of a developing (growing) long bone.

Epiphysis: The end (proximal or distal) of a long bone.

Epitheliochorial placenta: A placenta with six tissue layers between the maternal and fetal blood streams.

Epithelioid cell: A cell that resembles an epithelial cell.

Epithelium: A cellular tissue that covers external surfaces or lines cavities.

Erectile tissue: A highly vascular tissue that allows for an increase in turgidity of the penis or clitoris.

Ergot: An epidermal thickening found on the posterior surface of a horse's foot at the level of the distal end of the metacarpal bone.

Erythrocyte: A red blood cell.

Estrous cycle: A cyclic event of a female nonprimate mammal involving changes in anatomic structure of reproductive organs, changes in physiologic condition, and changes in sexual behavior.

Estrus: That segment of the estrous cycle during which the female is sexually receptive of the male.

Euchromatic: The relatively pale appearance of the nucleus of a fixed and stained cell when the chromatin is not highly coiled.

Exocrine gland: A gland with a duct system that carries a secretion to a body surface or cavity.

External auditory meatus: The canal of the external ear.

External ear: That portion of the ear external to the tympanic membrane, including the external auditory meatus and the pinna.

External elastic membrane: The elastic membrane external to the tunica media of some arteries.

External root sheath: The layer of cells in the wall of a hair follicle between the inner root sheath and the connective tissue sheath.

Eyelid: The movable, muscular fold covering the eye.

Fascicle: A bundle of structures such as a bundle of axons or a bundle of muscle cells.

Feather follicle: The epidermal structure from which a feather grows.

Feather pulp: The vascularized, mesenchyme-like tissue in the center of a developing feather.

Feather sheath: The thin, epidermal surface layer of the calamus of a growing feather. It eventually disintegrates except for a collarlike remnant around the calamus.

Fibroblasts: Ubiquitous cells of the connective tissue, responsible for producing the precursors of collagen and elastin and for producing the amorphous ground substance.

Fibroelastic tissue: Connective tissue proper containing a mixture of collagenous and elastic fibers.

Fibrous cartilage: Dense connective tissue containing isolated groups of chondrocytes surrounded by small amounts of matrix.

Fibrous tapetum lucidum: A reflective layer of the choroid of the eyes of horses and ruminants that is composed of collagenous fibers and fibroblasts.

Fibrous tunic: An external sheath comprised of fibers of connective tissue.

Filiform papilla: An outgrowth on the surface of the tongue bearing threadlike projections or spines.

Filoplume: A small, hairlike feather.

Filtration angle: In the eye the angle formed between the limbus, ciliary body, and the base of the iris.

Fixative: A chemical or mixture of chemicals used to preserve the structural characteristics of fresh tissue.

Foliate papilla: One of several foldlike elevations of the surface of the tongue.

Follicular tonsil: A tonsil with deep invaginations (crypts) of its surface epithelium.

Forestomach: The nonglandular portion of the stomach of the horse, ruminant, or pig.

Formed elements: Collectively, the erythrocytes, leukocytes, and platelets of the blood.

Fornix of conjunctiva: The point of reflection of the bulbar and palpebral conjunctiva.

Fossa: A cavity or a pit.

Fourth ventricle: The fluid-filled cavity of the medulla oblongata of the brain.

Frog: A caudal wedge-shaped part of the horse's hoof that lies between the bars.

Fundic gland region: A portion of the glandular stomach lying between the cardiac and pyloric gland regions.

Fungiform papilla: A mushroom-shaped elevation of the surface of the tongue.

Gallbladder: A saclike diverticulum of the common bile duct; functions as a storage depot for bile.

Ganglion cell layer (retina): Layer of cell bodies of neurons between the inner, plexiform layer and the nerve fiber layer.

Gastric furrow: A depression in the mucosa of the glandular stomach lined by columnar surface mucous cells.

Gastric pit (foveola): An invagination of the mucosa of the glandular stomach lined by columnar, surface mucous cells.

Germinal center: The central region of an activated lymphatic nodule, consisting mainly of lymphocytes of medium to large size.

Germinal epithelium: The epithelial layer covering the cortex of the ovary; composed of cuboidal or flattened cells.

Germinal vesicle: The nucleus of an oocyte.

Germinal zone (lens of eye): A band of epithelial cells located around the equator of the lens, capable of dividing throughout adult life.

Gingiva: The gum surrounding a tooth.

Glands of Moll: Sweat glands of the skin of the eyelids.

Glands of the anal sac: Tubular glands in the wall of an anal sac.

Glands of Zeiss: Sebaceous glands of the skin of the eyelids.

Glandular stomach: The portion of the stomach characterized by the presence of various types of tubular glands. It includes cardiac, fundic, body, and pyloric regions.

Globular (Globule) leukocyte: A leukocyte-like cell with large, round, eosinophilic granules, found in the mucosa of the intestine and stomach and reported to be derived from mast cell precursor cells in ruminants and rats.

Glomerular epithelium: The layer of podocytes in intimate contact with the glomerular capillary loops of a renal corpuscle.

Glomerulus: The tuft of capillary loops in the center of a renal corpuscle positioned between the afferent and efferent arteriole.

Glycogen body: A structure, centrally located in the spinal cord of birds, whose cells contain a central mass of glycogen.

Goblet cell: A mucus-secreting cell having the shape of a goblet.

Gonocyte: A primordial germ cell.

Granulocyte: A leukocyte having specific granules, e.g., eosinophil, neutrophil, basophil, and heterophil.

Granulosa lutein cell: The principal cell type of the corpus luteum; derived from a membrana granulosa cell of a postovulatory follicle.

Gray matter: That portion of the brain and spinal cord containing the cell bodies of neurons and mainly unmyelinated neuronal fibers.

Ground substance: The substance, consisting mainly of glycoproteins and glycosaminoglycans, that fills the spaces between the cellular and fibrous elements of connective tissue.

Guttural pouch: A diverticulum of the eustachian tubes of the horse.

H&E: Hematoxylin and eosin.

H band: A pale zone, devoid of actin filaments, located at the center of an A band of a sarcomere.

Hair bulb: The expanded base of a hair follicle.

Hair follicle: A derivative of the epidermis from which one or more hairs grow.

Hair matrix: That portion of a hair bulb where cell division occurs giving rise to a hair shaft

Hard keratin: A tough form of keratin found in hair and nails, among other places; contains more disulfide bonds and cystine than soft keratin.

Harderian gland: A large tubular gland that lies on the dorsal posterior surface of the eye.

Hassall's corpuscle: Acidophilic, concentric arrangements of reticular cells found in the medulla of the thymus of mammals.

Haversian canal: The canal in the center of a haversian system; contains blood vessels and nerves.

Haversian system (osteon): Collectively, concentrically arranged bony lamellae, osteocytes, and a haversian canal and its contents.

Head of the epididymis: The initial portion of the epididymis.

Helicine artery: A tortuous vessel that supplies blood to the cavernous spaces of the penis.

Helicotrema: A tiny opening at the apex of the cochlear canal of the inner ear connecting the cavity of the scala vestibuli with the cavity of the scala tympani.

Hemal node: A nodular structure found along blood vessels in ruminants; contains blood-filled sinuses between cellular cords.

Hematoma: Blood that has escaped from a blood vessel(s) within a tissue or organ.

Hemolymph node: A nodular structure, containing lymphatic vessels, whose sinuses receive a mixture of blood and lymph.

Henle's loop: The U-shaped portion of a nephron located between its proximal and distal convoluted tubules.

Hepatocyte: A liver cell.

Hepatoid gland: The nonsebaceous portion of the circumanal glands of the dog. Its cells resemble hepatocytes, hence the name hepatoid.

Herbst corpuscle: A tactile, encapsulated nerve ending of the skin of birds resembling the pacinian corpuscle but smaller.

Herring body: A neurosecretion found within the axons of unmyelinated neurosecretory cells of the hypothalamo-hypophyseal tract.

Heterochromatic: The appearance of the nucleus of a fixed and stained cell whose chromatin is tightly coiled. Such chromatin stains readily, resulting in a grainy nucleus.

Heterophil: The most abundant of the granulocytes of the chicken. Its specific granules are spindle-shaped and sometimes possess a distinct, ruby-red, spheric granule centrally.

Hilus: An invaginated region of the margin of an organ where blood vessels enter and leave.

Hilus cell: A group of epithelioid cells that may be found close to the rete ovarii near the hilus of the ovary in some mammals.

Histiocyte: A synonym for macrophage.

Holocrine secretion: A mode of secretion where disintegrated secretory cells and their product are released from a gland.

Hoof: The keratinized, epidermal, digital outgrowth of an ungulate.

Horn: A keratinized, epidermal outgrowth, with a bony core, of the head of some mammals.

Horn tubule (tubular horn): A tapering, keratinized, epidermal structure of the equine hoof that extends toward the surface from a dermal papilla.

Hyaline cartilage: The most common form of cartilage whose matrix has the appearance of ground glass in the fresh state.

Hypothalamohypophyseal tract: Collectively, the axons of neurosecretory cells within the infundibular stalk and infundibular process of the pituitary gland.

I band: That portion of adjacent sarcomeres lying to either side of the Z-line of an uncontracted myofibril. The I band contains actin myofilaments exclusively.

Immature bone: A highly cellular form of bone that becomes replaced by mature bone during development.

Incus: The ossicle of the middle ear located between the malleus and stapes.

Indeciduate placenta: A placenta whose endometrium and chorioallantoic membrane are in contact but do not fuse, seen in the mare, ruminants, and the sow.

Infundibular cavity: An extension of the third ventricle into the infundibular stalk of the pituitary and, in some animals, into the infundibular process.

Infundibular stalk: That portion of the neurohypophysis between the median eminence and the infundibular process.

Infundibulum: A ventral outpocketing of the diencephalon that develops into the neurohypophysis of the pituitary gland. Also, that part of the oviduct having a funnel shape and lying closest to the ovary.

Inner limiting membrane: The part of the photosensitive retina of the eye abutting the vitreous body.

Inner nuclear layer: The part of the photosensitive retina of the eye lying between the outer and inner plexiform layers.

Inner plexiform layer: The part of the photosensitive retina of the eye lying between the inner nuclear and ganglion cell layer.

Inner root sheath: That portion of a hair follicle lying between the hair and the external root sheath.

Inner tunnel: A large cavity lying within the organ of Corti of the inner ear.

Intercalated disc: A cell-surface modification found at both ends of cardiac muscle cells that is responsible for cell-to-cell adhesion and physiologic exchanges.

Intercalated duct: That part of the duct system of many glands that connects directly to the secretory unit.

Intermediate cell: An epithelial cell of the vagina with round corners, but larger than a parabasal cell, that occurs during the estrous cycle.

Internal ear: That part of the ear comprised of the semicircular ducts in semicircular canals, saccule and utricle in the vestibule, and the cochlea.

Internal elastic membrane: A sheetlike elastic membrane forming the outer boundary of the tunica intima of many arteries.

Interstitial cell (Leydig cell): A cell that produces testosterone and is found in the connective tissue between seminiferous tubules of the testes.

Interstitial gland cells: Epithelioid cells, arranged as cords, in the stroma of the ovaries of bitches and queens but not ordinarily found in other domestic mammals.

Interstitial system: A remnant of a preexisting haversian system of bone.

Interterritorial matrix: The matrix of hyaline cartilage surrounding the territorial matrix and possessing lesser concentrations of glycosaminoglycans than territorial matrix.

Intertubular horn: The keratinized epidermis of the hoof that surrounds the tubular horn.

Intralobular: That which is located within a lobule of a gland.

Intralobular duct: A duct located within the lobule of a gland.

Intramembranous bone: Bone that develops directly within or under a membrane of connective tissue.

Iris: The pigmented portion of the uvea surrounding the pupil of the eye.

Islet of Langerhans: A multicellular, endocrine structure embedded within the exocrine pancreas that produces insulin, glucagon, pancreatic polypeptide hormone, and somatostatin.

Isthmus (of the oviduct): The section of the oviduct attached to the uterus.

Isthmus (of the uropygial gland): The part of the drainage system of the uropygial gland located between the primary duct and the nipple.

Juxtaglomerular apparatus: A trinity of cellular structures associated with a nephron and consisting of the macula densa, juxtaglomerular cells, and mesangial cells.

Juxtaglomerular cell: A modified cell (smooth muscle) of an afferent arteriole of the kidney.

Keratinized: A structure whose cells have become filled with the protein keratin.

Keratinoid: A tough proteinaceous substance lining the gizzard of the chicken.

Keratohyalin granules: Vesicles found within the cells of the stratum granulosum of the epidermis whose contents will form the amorphous portion of keratin.

Köhler illumination: Bright, even illumination required for optimal light microscopy and achieved by adjusting the light source in a prescribed manner

Krause's gland: An accessory lacrimal gland that may be either serous or mixed.

Kupffer cell: A macrophage located within the blood vascular system of the liver.

l.s.: Longitudinal section.

Labia: Lips.

Labial gland: Mixed glands found within the lips of the mouth.

Labyrinth: A complicated structural arrangement.

Lacrimal gland: The tear gland.

Lacuna: A small cavity or space.

Lagena: A terminal expansion of the cochlear duct of the inner ear of birds.

Lamella: A layer of material, e.g., of bone.

Lamina cribrosa: The sievelike part of the sclera that partitions groups of axons of the optic nerve.

Lamina propria: The loose connective tissue beneath the epithelium of a mucous membrane.

Lamina subglandularis: A thick sheet of collagenous fibers (stratum compactum) and the accompanying layer of fibroblasts (stratum granulosum) between the base of the glands and the muscularis mucosae of the stomach of the cat and sometimes the dog. The lamina may also occur in the small intestine of carnivores.

Laminar region: The part of the wall of the hoof that is composed of numerous plates (laminae) that function to suspend the third phalanx from the hoof.

Layer of rods and cones: In the retina of the eye, the layer comprised of the dendrites of the photoreceptor cells.

Lens: A biconvex, transparent structure comprised of lens fibers, positioned between the iris and the vitreous body.

Lens body: The part of the eye of the chicken, exclusive of the annular pad, whose lens fibers are oriented parallel to the optical axis of the eye.

Lens epithelium: The layer of simple cuboidal epithelium on the anterior surface (iris side) of the lens.

Lens fibers: Transparent, elongated, prismatic cells forming the bulk of the substance of the lens of the eye.

Leukocyte: A white blood cell, either granulocyte or agranulocyte.

Light cell: Any cell, among contrasting dark cells, with pale cytoplasm; found in such places as the epithelium of the gallbladder or the tegmentum vasculosum of the inner ear of the chicken, among other places.

Light zone (of the glandular stomach): The initial portion of the fundic gland region of the stomach of a carnivore; compared with the dark zone of the fundic gland region, it is shorter and its mucosa is thinner.

Limbus: The boundary line between the cornea and sclera.

Lobule: The subdivision of a lobe of an organ such as a gland or the lung.

Loop of Henle: The U-shaped portion of a nephron joining a proximal and distal convoluted tubule.

Loose (areolar) connective tissue: A type of connective tissue proper whose fibers are in the form of a noncompacted, open meshwork.

Luteal cells (interstitial cells): The lutein cells of the corpus luteum of the mammalian ovary, or the pale interstitial cells within the theca externa surrounding the oocyte of an ovarian follicle of the chicken.

Lymph node: A lymphatic organ having both afferent and efferent lymphatic vessels.

Lymphatic nodule: A temporary, spherical, or oval structure, consisting of numerous lymphocytes, found within various lymphatic organs; may also be found anywhere within the loose connective tissue of the body.

Lymphocyte: An agranulocyte with scant cytoplasm and, typically, a large, round, or broadly oval nucleus.

Macrophage: A phagocytic cell, derived from a monocyte, and widely distributed in tissues and organs throughout the body.

Macula (of the ear): A patch of sensory and supporting cells found within the sacculus (saccule) and utriculus (utricle) of the inner ear.

Macula densa: A part of the juxtaglomerular apparatus of a nephron and formed from closely packed epithelial cells of a portion of the wall of the distal convoluted tubule.

Magnum: The part of the chicken's oviduct whose gland cells produce the albumin of the egg.

Malleus: The middle ear ossicle in contact with the tympanic membrane.

Mammary gland: The milk-producing organ of the mammalian female.

Marginal zone: Splenic tissue located between the white and red pulp.

Mast cell: A large, granular, ubiquitous cell of the connective tissue that produces histamine.

Mature bone: Bone with an acidophilic matrix and fewer osteocytes than the immature bone it replaces during development.

Median eminence: The region of the floor of the diencephalon of the brain from which the infundibular stalk of the pituitary arises.

Medulla: The inner region of an organ such as the medulla of the kidney, ovary or lymph node.

Medullary cone: The cone-shaped medullary portion of the chicken's kidney that contains segments of uriniferous tubules.

Medullary cord: One of many interconnected segments of diffuse connective tissue, surrounded by medullary sinuses, within the medulla of a lymph node.

Medullary nephron: The larger of two forms of nephrons of the chicken's kidney having the characteristics of the mammalian nephron.

Medullary sinuses: The lymph-filled spaces surrounding the medullary cords of a lymph node.

Megakaryocyte: An extraordinarily large cell of the bone marrow that produces blood platelets by a budding process and releases them directly into the sinusoids of the marrow.

Meissner's plexus: As seen in histologic section, a spindle-shaped collection of parasympathetic neurons and their processes found within the submucosa of the digestive tract.

Melanocyte: A large, branched cell that produces melanosomes (tiny vesicles containing pigment).

Membrana granulosa: The cells that line the antrum of a mammalian ovarian follicle.

Membranous labyrinth: The hollow, soft-tissue structures of the inner ear, i.e., cochlear duct, utriculus, sacculus, and semicircular ducts.

Merkel's cell: A cell of the epidermis of the skin that has contact with tactile nerve endings.

Merocrine gland: An exocrine gland whose secretory cells release droplets of secretion by exocytosis.

Mesangial cells: Phagocytic cells found within the renal glomerulus.

Mesenchyme: Embryonal connective tissue that consists of stellate mesenchyme cells and ground substance.

Mesobronchus: The intrapulmonary, primary bronchus of the chicken's lung.

Mesometrium: The mesentery supporting the uterus from the abdominal wall.

Mesosalpinx: The mesentery supporting the oviduct from the abdominal wall.

Mesothelium: The mesodermally derived, simple squamous epithelium, covering the surface of mesenteries and organs that protrude into coelomic cavities of the body.

Metachromsia: The circumstance in which a cell or tissue component acquires a color different from the dye solution with which it is stained.

Metamyelocyte: A developing granulocyte that possesses an indented nucleus and specific granules.

Metestrus: That part of the estrous cycle between estrus and diestrus. The development of the corpus luteum occurs during metestrus.

Microplacentome: A placental structure of the mare consisting of a small tuft of chorionic villi and a crypt of the endometrium into which it is inserted.

Middle ear: A subdivision of the ear comprised of three small ossicles (malleus, incus, and stapes) or of a columella.

Mixed gland: An exocrine gland whose secretory units consist of either mucous or serous cells or of a combination of these cells. Or, a gland with both endocrine and exocrine components.

Modiolus: The pillarlike bone in the center of the cochlea.

Monocyte: A large, agranular leukocyte with an oval, indented or horseshoe-shaped nucleus and pale, blue-gray, often vacuolated, cytoplasm.

Mucosa: In the digestive tract, the mucous membrane comprised of an epithelium, lamina propria, and muscularis mucosae (latter is lacking in the mouth, pharynx, and portions of the esophagus). In other organ systems, the epithelium lining the organ together with the underlying lamina propria constitutes the mucosa.

Mucous acinus: The bulblike secretory unit of a gland whose cells secrete mucus.

Mucous connective tissue: A form of embryonal connective tissue consisting of amorphous ground substance, loosely arranged collagenous fibers, and fibroblasts.

Mucous membrane: A synonym for mucosa.

Mucous neck cell: A cell of the neck region of a gastric gland that produces mucus.

Multilaminar primary follicle: A preantral ovarian follicle whose oocyte is surrounded by several layers of follicle cells.

Multilocular adipose cell: An adipocyte whose lipid content is located within numerous, small vesicles.

Multinucleate giant cell: A large, phagocytic cell with many nuclei; formed by the coalescence of macrophages.

Multipolar neuron: A nerve cell having numerous dendrites and a single axon.

Muscularis externa: The outermost layers of muscle in the wall of the digestive tract; may be smooth muscle, skeletal muscle, or both.

Muscularis mucosae: The layer (s) of smooth muscle below the lamina propria of the mucosa of the digestive tract.

Myelin sheath: A derivative of the cell membrane of a Schwann cell or of a oligodendrocyte; the sheath is arranged in concentric layers around axons.

Myeloblast: An early stage in the development of a granulocyte of the bone marrow.

Myelocyte: The developmental stage of a granulocyte following the promyelocyte stage.

Myocardium: The middle, muscular tunic of the heart wall.

Myoepithelial cell: An epithelial cell with contractile properties, as found on the surface of many glandular secretory units; also, one of the many contractile cells forming the iridial dilator of the eye.

Myofibril: One of many contractile units, formed from linearly joined sarcomeres, as in skeletal and cardiac muscle cells.

Myoid cell: A contractile cell, such as found at the surface of a seminiferous tubule.

Myometrium: The layers of smooth muscle external to the endometrium of the uterus.

Nasal cavity: One of a pair of bilaterally arranged chambers located between the external nares and nasopharynx.

Nasolabial gland: An exocrine gland of the subcutis of the planum nasolabiale of ruminants.

Nasopharynx: That portion of the pharynx between the internal nares and the oropharynx.

Necrotic: Pertaining to dead cells or tissue.

Nephron: The portion of a uriniferous tubule before the collecting tubule; includes the renal corpuscle, proximal convoluted tubule, loop of Henle, and the distal convoluted tubule.

Nerve fiber layer (of the retina): The portion of the retina between the ganglion cell layer and the inner limiting membrane; consists of axons of ganglion cells.

Neurilemma: The covering (sheath), formed from Schwann cells or oligodendrocytes, of a nerve cell's process. The neurilemma may or may not include a myelin component.

Neuroglia: Supportive cells of the central nervous system; considered to be about ten times more numerous than neurons.

Neurohypophysis: The portion of the pituitary gland that is derived from the infundibulum; consists of the median eminence, infundibular stalk, and infundibular process (pars nervosa).

Neuromuscular spindle: A fusiform-shaped proprioceptive structure within the skeletal musculature.

Neutrophil: A polymorphonuclear granulocyte with fine specific granules.

Nictitating membrane: The third eyelid found in some animals.

Nissl granule: The rough endoplasmic reticulum of a neuron.

Nonglandular stomach: The part of the stomach lacking glandular elements.

Nonsinusal spleen: A type of spleen having poorly developed sinuses or no sinuses, as found in the cat, horse, pig, and ruminants.

Nuclear bag fiber: An intrafusal fiber (modified skeletal muscle cell) of a neuromuscular spindle, characterized by the presence of many closely packed nuclei.

Nucleolus: A small round or oval structure, within the nucleus of a cell, where ribonucleoprotein is synthesized.

Odontoblasts: Cells on the surface of dental papillae that produce uncalcified dentin (predentin).

Olfactory epithelium: The pseudostratified columnar epithelium of the nasal cavity that is comprised of sensory cells, supporting cells, and basal cells.

Omasum: The third subdivision of the ruminant forestomach.

Optic disc: The portion of the eye where the axons of the nerve fiber layer of the retina converge to form the optic nerve. There are no light sensitive cells present in the disc, hence the name blind spot.

Optic nerve: The second cranial nerve.

Ora ciliaris retinae: The point of transition from the photosensitive to the nonphotosensitive part of the retina.

Organ of Corti: The part of the inner ear that is sensitive to sound.

Oropharynx: The portion of the pharynx that is located behind the mouth.

Orthochromatophilic erythroblast: In the erythroid line, the smallest nucleated cell.

Os penis: A bone within the glans of the penis of carnivores.

Osseous spiral lamina: A spiral shelf of bone around the modiolus of the cochlea.

Osteoblast: A cell that synthesizes and secretes bone matrix.

Osteoclast: A multinucleate giant cell that resorbs bone matrix.

Osteocyte: A mature bone cell.

Osteoid: Uncalcified bone matrix.

Otolith: A tiny structure with a prismatic shape found embedded in the gelatinous covering (otolithic membrane) of a macula of the utricle and saccule of the inner ear.

Otolithic membrane: The gelatinous covering of a macula of the utricle and saccule of the inner ear.

Outer enamel epithelium: A layer of cells abutting (externally) the stellate reticulum of a developing fetal tooth.

Outer limiting membrane: The retinal layer formed from the plasma membranes of Müller cells and located between the layer of rods and cones and the outer nuclear layer.

Outer nuclear layer: The retinal layer consisting of the nuclei of the rod and cone cells.

Outer plexiform layer: The retinal layer composed of neuronal fibers and located between the outer nuclear layer and the inner plexiform layer.

Outer root sheath (external root sheath): The layer of cells in the wall of a hair follicle between the inner root sheath and the connective tissue sheath.

Ovarian follicle: The cellular unit surrounding an oocyte in the ovary.

Oviduct: The tubular organ that receives an oocyte from the ovary and conveys it, after fertilization, to the exterior (birds) or to the uterus (mammals, except prototherians) for implantation.

Oxyphil: A parenchymal cell of the parathyroid gland.

Pacinian corpuscle: An encapsulated nerve ending that responds to heavy pressure as opposed to light touch.

Palpebral conjunctiva: The mucous membrane lining the eyelid.

Paneth cell: A secretory cell whose acidophilic granules contain lysozyme; found in the intestinal glands of some mammals.

Papillary duct: A large urinary duct that opens to the renal pelvis from the tip of a renal papilla of the kidney.

Papillary layer: The upper layer of the dermis with finger-like extensions (called dermal papillae) into the epidermis of thick skin.

Parabasal cell: A sloughed, small, round vaginal epithelial cell, found in vaginal smears taken from an animal in anestrus.

Parabronchus (tertiary bronchus): An intrapulmonary branch of a secondary bronchus of the chicken lung.

Parafollicular cell (C cell): A large, pale cell found between epithelial cells of thyroid follicles and also between follicles; produces the hormone calcitonin whose action lowers blood calcium level.

Parenchyma cells: The cells responsible for the special function of an organ as opposed to the organ's stroma (framework of connective tissue).

Parietal cell: A large acidophilic cell of the fundic and pyloric gland regions of the stomach that produces hydrochloric acid.

Pars ciliaris retinae: The bilayered, nonphotosensitive portion of the retina associated with the ciliary body and located between the ora ciliaris retinae and the pars iridica retinae.

Pars convoluta (cortical labyrinth): That part of the renal cortex that contains renal corpuscles and convoluted tubules, and is located between medullary rays.

Pars disseminata: The scattered portions of the prostate gland.

Pars distalis: Derived from Rathke's pouch and the largest component of the pituitary gland. Alone or with the pars tuberalis, called the anterior lobe of the pituitary.

Pars intermedia: That part of the pituitary gland located between the pars distalis and pars nervosa. A derivative of Rathke's pouch.

Pars iridica retinae: That part of the nonphotosensitive retina located on the side of the iris facing the lens.

Pars nervosa: The major part of the neurohypophysis and a derivative of the hypothalamus; with the pars intermedia, forms the posterior lobe of the pituitary.

Pars radiata (medullary or cortical rays): The part of the renal cortex alternating with the pars convoluta and consisting of collecting tubules and the straight portions of nephrons.

Pars tuberalis: The part of the pituitary gland that forms a collar around the infundibular stalk; derived from Rathke's pouch.

Pecten: A thin, vascular, pleated membrane that protrudes from the ventral surface of the chicken's eye into the cavity of the vitreous body.

Pectinate ligament (uveal meshwork): A loose network of elastic fibers, covered by squamous cells, that spans the filtration angle of the eye.

Penicillus: Term applied to the pulp arteries of the spleen and their branches because, collectively, they resemble the bristles of an artist's brush.

Penis, body of: Shaft of the intromittent organ of the male.

Penis, glans of: The expanded terminal end of the penis.

Periarterial lymphatic sheath: The white pulp of the spleen.

Pericardium: The visceral and parietal serosa of the pericardial cavity.

Perichondrium: The chondrogenic, dense irregular connective tissue covering of hyaline or elastic cartilage.

Perilymph: The fluid found in the bony labyrinth of the inner ear surrounding the membranous labyrinth.

Perimetrium: The serosa of the uterus.

Perimysium: The connective tissue surrounding a fascicle of muscle cells.

Perineurium: The connective tissue surrounding a bundle of nerve cell fibers (axons, dendrites, or both).

Periople: The proximal border of the horse's hoof.

Periosteum: The osteogenic, dense irregular connective tissue that covers portions of many bones.

Peritoneum: The serosa lining a coelomic cavity.

Perivitelline membrane: The membrane abutting the cell membrane of the oocyte of a chicken's ovarian follicle.

Pessulus: A small bone supporting the syrinx of a chicken.

Peyer's patch: An aggregation of lymphatic tissue (nodular and diffuse) in the lamina propria and submucosa of the small intestine, especially the ileum.

Photosensitive retina: The portion of the retina containing light sensitive rod and cone cells.

Pia mater: The delicate, well vascularized meninx in contact with the surface of the brain.

Pigment epithelium: The pigmented layer of cells forming the outermost boundary of the retina.

Pineal gland: A dorsal evagination from the roof of the diencephalon of the brain.

Pinealocytes: The epithelioid, acidophilic, parenchymal cells of the pineal gland.

Pinna (auricle): The sound-collecting auricular appendage of the head.

Pituicytes: Neuroglial cells located among the neuronal fibers of the pars nervosa of the pituitary gland.

Placenta: A nutritive organ, derived in part from both the endometrium and the chorion.

Placentome: A structure formed from a cotyledon (clump of chorionic villi) and caruncle (elevation of the endometrium) of a cotyledonary placenta.

Planum: The flat surface of skin located between the external nares.

Plasma: The acellular fluid portion of circulating blood.

Plasma cell: A derivative of the B cell that synthesizes immunoglobulins.

Platelet: A fragment of membrane-bound cytoplasm, derived by budding from a megakaryocyte, with an important role in blood clotting.

Plexus: A localized network of any of the following: neurons and their processes, blood vessels, or lymphatic vessels.

Plica: A fold.

Podocyte: A highly branched cell whose processes interdigitate with those of other podocytes to form the glomerular epithelium of the Bowman's capsule of the kidney.

Polychromatophilic erythroblast: An erythroblast of medium size with cytoplasm exhibiting both basophilic and acidophilic areas.

Polymorphonuclear leukocyte: A granulocyte with a segmented nucleus.

Portal tract (area): An aggregation of blood vessels (and sometimes lymphatic vessels) and a bile ductule within the interlobular connective tissue of the liver.

Postcapillary venule: A venule, of the deep cortex of a lymph node, whose endothelial cells are cuboidal.

Posterior chamber (of the eye): The cavity, containing aqueous humor, that is located between the iris and the lens.

Posterior epithelium (of the cornea): The simple cuboidal or squamous epithelium covering the side of the cornea in contact with the aqueous humor.

Preantral follicle: A growing ovarian follicle that has not yet formed an antrum.

Predentin: Uncalcified dentin.

Prepuce: The foreskin of the penis.

Primary bronchus: A large bronchus branching directly from the trachea.

Primary follicle: An ovarian follicle whose oocyte is surrounded by a single layer of cuboidal cells. The term is also used, by some authors, for a multilaminar follicle.

Primary hair: A large hair shaft produced by a compound follicle.

Primary spermatocyte: A diploid cell formed by differentiation from a spermatogonium.

Primordial follicle: The earliest, smallest, and most numerous of ovarian follicles; consists of an oocyte surrounded by a layer of flat follicle cells.

Principal cell (chief cell): A parenchymal cell of the parathyroid gland. The name is also used for the small, basophilic cell of the glandular stomach that secretes pepsinogen.

Proctodeum: That part of the chicken's cloaca that joins the large intestine.

Proerythrocyte (rubriblast): A large, round cell of the erythroid line with basophilic cytoplasm and a large round nucleus.

Proestrus: The first stage of the estrous cycle; characterized by growth of the endometrium.

Promyelocyte: An early granulocyte, recognized by a large nucleus with nucleoli and azurophilic cytoplasmic granules.

Prostate gland: An accessory male reproductive gland whose secretion contributes to the seminal fluid at ejaculation.

Proventriculus: The glandular portion of the stomach of the chicken.

Proximal convoluted tubule: The long, highly convoluted tubule of a nephron that arises from a renal corpuscle and whose cells have a distinctive brush border.

Pseudostratified epithelium: An epithelium that appears to be stratified but is not. All of its cells are in contact with the basement membrane. Its stratified appearance is the result of its cells being of different heights and their nuclei being located at different levels.

Pulp artery: An artery within the red pulp of the spleen that arises from the central artery of the periarterial lymphatic sheath

Pupil: The opening in the center of the iris.

Purkinje cell: A large, modified cardiac muscle cell that forms a part of the heart's conduction system. The word also identifies the large multipolar nerve cells present in the cerebellum at the junction of the granular and molecular layers.

Pyknotic cell: A cell with a shrunken, basophilic nucleus or a cell that has become reduced in size.

Pyloric gland region: The terminal glandular region of the stomach, characterized by deep gastric pits and mucous glands with some parietal cells.

Pyramidal cell: A nerve cell having the shape of a pyramid, as found in the cerebral cortex.

Rachis: The part of the central shaft of a contour feather bearing the vanes.

Rathke's pouch: An ectodermal diverticulum from the roof of the oral cavity of an embryo.

Red pulp: The portion of the parenchyma of the spleen other than the white pulp; characterized by the abundance of erythrocytes.

Renal corpuscle: A component of the nephron consisting of Bowman's capsule and the glomerulus.

Renal cortex: The outer part of the kidney, identified by the presence of numerous renal corpuscles.

Renal medulla: The region of the kidney internal to the cortex and dominated by loops of Henle, collecting tubules, and vasa rectae.

Renal papilla: The tip of a renal pyramid.

Renal pelvis: The expanded end of the ureter located within the hilus of the kidney.

Respiratory bronchiole: A bronchiole with scattered alveoli within its walls and positioned between a terminal bronchiole and an alveolar duct.

Rete ovarii: Channels, lined by cuboidal cells, located within the medulla of the ovaries of carnivores and ruminants.

Rete testis: A network of channels located within the loose connective tissue of the mediastinum testis.

Reticular fiber: A thin, argyrophilic, collagenous fiber

Reticular layer (of dermis): The dense irregular connective tissue layer of the dermis.

Reticular structure: A diffuse form of Hassall's corpuscle in the thymus of the chicken, consisting of an irregular mass of reticular cells, including degenerating ones, in the medulla of lobules.

Reticular tissue: A special form of connective tissue proper consisting of a feltwork of reticular fibers functioning as a supportive framework for cells of the parenchyma. Among other locations, it is well represented in the liver, spleen, and bone marrow.

Reticulocyte: A newly produced erythrocyte.

Retina (photosensitive): The part of the retinal tunic of the eye containing light sensitive rod and cone cells.

Retinal tunic: The innermost layer of the wall of the eye, consisting of the photosensitive retina, the pars ciliaris retinae, and the pars iridica retinae.

Romanovsky stain: A compound dye substance used for staining the various different cells of the blood and bone marrow.

Rouleaux: An arrangement of erythrocytes, in a smear preparation, resembling a stack of discs or coins.

Rumen: The largest subdivision of the forestomach of ruminants.

Sacculus (saccule): A part of the membranous labyrinth within the vestibule of the inner ear; contains a macula whose sensory cells, when stimulated, make an animal aware of the position of its head in space and the sensations of linear acceleration and deceleration.

Sarcolemma: The plasmalemma (cell membrane) of a muscle cell.

Sarcomere: The unit of contraction of a skeletal or cardiac muscle myofibril; every sarcomere of a myofibril is located between adjacent Z lines.

Sarcoplasm: The cytoplasm of a muscle cell.

Satellite cell: A neuroglia cell in close proximity to the cell body of a neuron. Also, a cell with mesenchymal properties found intimately associated with skeletal muscle cells.

Scala tympani: A chamber of the inner ear, filled with perilymph, and lying below the floor of the cochlear duct.

Scala vestibuli: A chamber of the inner ear, filled with perilymph and lying above the roof (vestibular membrane) of the cochlear duct.

Schiff's reagent: A colorless fuchsin sulfurous acid (leucofuchsin) solution. Leucofuchsin is used in the Periodic Acid-Schiff (PAS) reaction for demonstrating the presence of complex carbohydrates, e.g., glycogen, starch, cellulose, and proteoglycans, among others.

Schwann cell: A cell of the peripheral nervous system closely associated with neuronal processes and responsible for forming the neurilemma.

Sclera: A part of the outermost tunic of the eye, consisting of dense irregular connective tissue.

Scleral cartilage: A cup-shaped layer of cartilage within the sclera of the eye of the chicken.

Scleral ossicle: A plate of bone, located anterior to the scleral cartilage, within the sclera of the eye of the chicken.

Scleral trabecular meshwork: A webwork of elastic and collagenous fibers, within the filtration angle of the eye of the chicken, whose spaces are continuous with the spaces of Fontana of the uveal meshwork (pectinate ligament).

Scleral venous plexus: A system of channels that drain excess aqueous humor away from the eye.

Sebaceous gland: A holocrine gland of the skin that produces an oily secretion.

Sebaceous zone: The sebaceous region of the uropygial gland of the chicken.

Secondary follicle: An ovarian follicle of the mammal with a C-shaped antrum

Secondary spermatocyte: The stage of spermatogenesis between primary spermatocyte and early spermatid.

Secretory duct: See striated duct.

Semicircular canal: The tubular channel of the inner ear within the temporal bone that contains a semicircular duct.

Seminal vesicle: An accessory reproductive gland that contributes to the seminal fluid at ejaculation.

Seminiferous tubule: A highly convoluted tubule within the testis where spermatogenesis occurs.

Sensory cell: A neuron that conveys sensory information to the central nervous system.

Sensory hair cells (ear): Cells, with stereocilia on their apical surfaces that, when stimulated, will initiate an impulse to the brain for interpretation; found in the organ of Corti, sacculus, utricle, and crista ampullaris.

Serosa: The lining membrane of the coelom in all its subdivisions; consists of a mesothelium and layer of underlying connective tissue.

Serous demilune: A crescent-shaped cap, as seen in histologic section, of serous cells on the surface of a mucous acinus.

Serous membrane: A synonym for serosa.

Sertoli cell: A large, multifunctional cell, forming part of the epithelium of the wall of a seminiferous tubule.

Serum: The acellular fluid part of blood obtained following coagulation.

Sex cord: A convoluted cord of cells, within the testis of an embryo or young animal, whose cells will differentiate into stem cells.

Sharpey's fibers: Collagenous fibers that anchor the periosteum to bone or a tendon to bone.

Sheathed artery: A vessel of the white pulp of the spleen of the chicken that is surrounded by a ring of reticular cells.

Shell gland: That portion of the oviduct of the chicken whose secretion produces the egg shell; the shell gland is also called the uterus.

Simple epithelium: An epithelium consisting of a single layer of cells, all of which are attached to the basement membrane.

Sinus hair: A tactile hair, limited to the facial region, that originates from a highly innervated follicle containing a large blood-filled sinus.

Sinusal spleen: A spleen whose red pulp is characterized by numerous, blood-filled sinuses.

Sinusoid: A thin-walled blood vessel with the characteristics of a capillary but having a larger and more irregular diameter.

Small artery: Arbitrarily, an artery with up to 8 or 9 layers of smooth muscle cells in the tunica media. The smallest of the small arteries is called an arteriole.

Smegma: The soft, cheesy deposit of desquamated epithelial cells and glandular secretions found on the glans and prepuce of the penis; it is also found in the urethral pouch of the stallion.

Smudged cell: A ruptured, or otherwise distorted, leukocyte found in a blood or bone marrow smear.

Soft keratin: A form of keratin, found in such places as the stratum corneum, that has fewer disulfide bonds and less cystine than hard keratin.

Spaces of Fontana: Cavities filled with aqueous humor within the trabecular meshworks of the eye.

Specific granules: Granules within the cytoplasm of a granulocyte that characterize the cell, e.g., eosinophilic granules of an eosinophil.

Sperm-host gland: Tubular glands of the vagina of the oviduct of the chicken that serve as storage depots for deposited sperm.

Spermatid: The haploid cell following the secondary spermatocyte during spermatogenesis.

Spermatogenic cell: Any precursor of a spermatozoon found within the seminiferous epithelium.

Spermatogonium: The most immature spermatogenic cell of the seminiferous epithelium

Sphincter (iris): The circumferentially arranged smooth muscle of the iris that enables pupillary constriction.

Spicule: A small, frequently irregularly-shaped, piece of bone.

Spiral ganglion: The auditory ganglion associated with the modiolus of the cochlea.

Spiral ligament: A thickening of the periosteal lining of the cochlear canal.

Spiral limbus: An elevation of connective tissue resting on the osseous spiral lamina of the cochlea.

Spiral tunnel: The space below the tectorial membrane of the inner ear.

Spleen: A major lymphatic and blood-filtering organ.

Spongy bone (cancellous bone): An architectural form of bone consisting of a three dimensional meshwork of bony trabeculae containing numerous marrow spaces.

Stapes: The middle ear ossicle attached to the oval window in the petrous portion of the temporal bone.

Stellate reticulum: A portion of the enamel organ of a developing tooth characterized by star-shaped cells.

Stereocilia: Long microvilli found on the apices of certain cells, e.g., on the epithelial cells lining portions of the duct of the epididymis and on the sensory hair cells of the inner ear.

Straight tubule: A tubule that connects a seminiferous tubule with the rete testis.

Stratified epithelium: An epithelium consisting of two or more layers of cells with only the basal layer being in contact with the basement membrane.

Stratum basale: The layer of cells in contact with the basement membrane of the epidermis.

Stratum cavernosum: The erectile tissue of the pelvic urethra.

Stratum compactum: A thick layer of collagenous fibers located between the base of the glands and the muscularis mucosae of the glandular stomach of the cat and some dogs.

Stratum corneum: The outermost, keratinized layer of the epidermis.

Stratum germinativum: The layers of the epidermis below the stratum corneum of the chicken, i.e., the basal, intermediate, and transitional layers. In mammals, stratum germinativum is a term sometimes employed to include both the stratum basale and the stratum spinosum.

Stratum granulosum: The layer of cells below the stratum corneum whose cytoplasm contains keratohyalin granules.

Stratum intermedium: The layer of cells located between ameloblasts and the stellate reticulum of a developing tooth.

Stratum lucidum: The layer of pale epidermal cells located between the stratum corneum and stratum granulosum of thick skin.

Stratum medium: The major portion of the wall of the horse's hoof, consisting of tubular and intertubular horn that extends from the coronary region to the surface of the ground.

Stratum spinosum: The layer of the epidermis directly above the stratum basale. It is characterized by cells whose membranes have shrunken in all places except where desmosomes occur, giving the cells the appearance of having spines.

Stratum vasculare: The richly vascularized and well innervated layer wedged between the inner circular and outer longitudinal layers of the myometrium of the bicornuate uterus of domestic mammals.

Stria vascularis: The stratified cuboidal epithelium of the side of the cochlear duct that is attached to the spiral ligament of the cochlear canal. Capillaries occur among the superficial cuboidal cells of the stria.

Striated border: The border of apical microvilli of intestinal epithelial cells as seen in profile view.

Striated duct: An intralobular duct of a salivary gland whose epithelial cells have vertical stripes (invaginations of the plasma membrane) along their basal ends.

Stroma (corneal): The predominant layer of the cornea; also called the substantia propria. It consists of lamellae of collagenous fibers oriented parallel to the corneal surface.

Subarachnoid space: A space, filled with cerebrospinal fluid, located between the arachnoid layer and pia mater of the brain and spinal cord.

Subcapsular sinus: The space, filled with lymph, beneath the capsule of a lymph node.

Subcutis (subcutaneous connective tissue): The layer of loose connective tissue deep to the skin.

Submucosa: The layer of connective tissue beneath a mucous membrane.

Sulcus (chicken proventriculus): A depression between folds of the mucosa of the proventriculus.

Superficial cell: Similar in size and shape to a superficial intermediate cell of a vaginal smear, but with a pyknotic nucleus, faded nucleus, or no nucleus.

Superficial gland of the nictitating membrane: Depending on the type of animal, a serous, mucous, or mixed gland surrounding the base of the cartilage supporting the membrane.

Superficial intermediate cell: A large, vaginal, epithelial cell with angular edges and a round nucleus found in vaginal smears.

Sweat gland: A tubular, or saclike gland of the skin; may be either apocrine or merocrine.

Syndesmochorial placenta: The type of placenta of ewes and nanny goats where five layers of tissue separate maternal from fetal blood.

Synovial fluid: The clear, lubricating fluid within the synovial cavity of a synovial joint.

Syntrophoblast: The syncytial outer layer of the trophoblast.

Syrinx: The voice box of the chicken, located where the trachea bifurcates into two bronchi.

Taenia ceci: Flat bands of smooth muscle and elastic fibers within the cecum of horses and pigs.

Taenia coli: Flat bands of smooth muscle and elastic fibers within the colon of horses and pigs.

Tail of the epididymis: The end of the epididymis that joins with the vas deferens.

Tapetum lucidum: A fibrous or cellular reflective layer of the choroid coat of the eye.

Tarsal glands: Large multilobular sebaceous glands located within the tarsus (plate of dense connective tissue) of the palpebral conjunctiva.

Tarsus: A plate of dense connective tissue within the eyelid. It is located between the dermis of the skin and the lamina propria of the palpebral conjunctiva.

Taste bud: A multicellular, barrel-shaped structure, consisting of sensory and supportive cells and located within various parts of the epithelium of the tongue.

Taste pore: A tiny opening at the tip of a taste bud.

Teat canal: A channel, lined by stratified squamous epithelium, that opens onto the tip of a teat.

Teat sinus: A channel, lined by a bistratified epithelium, that opens into a teat canal.

Tectorial membrane: A proteinaceous membrane that overlies and contacts the stereocilia of the sensory cells of the organ of Corti of the inner ear.

Tegmentum vasculosum: A vascularized membrane separating the cochlear duct from the overlying scala vestibuli of the inner ear of the chicken.

Tendon: A bundle or band of dense regular connective tissue connecting a muscle to a bone.

Tendon sheath: A layer of cells and fibers of connective tissue on the surface of a tendon.

Territorial matrix: The matrix, rich in sulfated glycosaminoglycans, immediately surrounding a chondrocyte (s) of hyaline cartilage.

Tertiary follicle: The large ovarian follicle just prior to ovulation; also called a Graafian follicle.

Theca externa: The outer (connective tissue) layer of the wall of a mammalian ovarian follicle.

Theca folliculi: A sheath of stromal cells, surrounding a growing, mammalian ovarian follicle, that will differentiate into a theca externa and theca interna.

Theca interna: The inner cellular and well vascularized layer of the wall of a mammalian ovarian follicle.

Theca lutein cell: A small lutein cell of a corpus luteum derived from a cell of the theca interna.

Thick skin: Hairless skin with an epidermis that is many cells thick, e.g., skin of a digital pad or of the planum nasolabiale.

Thin skin: Skin with an epidermis that is only a few cells thick; e.g., skin of the trunk or of the legs among other places.

Thrombocyte: A blood cell of the chicken with a role in blood clot formation.: Also, incorrectly used as a synonym for a platelet of mammals.

Thyroid follicle: A vesicle of the thyroid gland, formed of a simple epithelium, that contains the storage form of thyroxin called thyroglobulin.

Tonsil: A lymphatic organ found below the epithelium in such places as the tongue and pharynx.

Trabecula: A part of the framework of connective tissue of an organ or structure, e.g., a bundle of fibers of the splenic stroma or any of the irregularly shaped pieces of bone that form part of the three dimensional latticework of spongy bone.

Transitional epithelium: An epithelium, limited to the urinary system, whose appearance depends on the amount of fluid pressure applied against it.

Trophoblast: The mesectodermal layer covering the blastocyst.

Tubuloacinar gland: A gland whose secretory units consist of tubules and acini.

Tunica adventitia: The outermost layer of connective tissue of a blood vessel.

Tunica albuginia: A layer of dense connective tissue surrounding a structure, e.g., the layer beneath the germinal epithelium of the ovary or the layer surrounding the testis.

Tunica intima: The innermost tunic of the wall of a blood vessel.

Tunica media: The middle, muscle layer of the wall of a blood vessel.

Tunica vaginalis: The serosa of the testis and the epididymis.

Tympanic cavity: The cavity containing the middle ear ossicles; also called the cavity of the middle ear.

Tympanic membrane (eardrum): The membrane between the external auditory meatus and the tympanic cavity (cavity of the middle ear).

Type I cell (of the macula): A chalice-shaped sensory cell of the epithelium of the macula of a sacculus

Unipolar neuron: A nerve cell with two processes that arise from a single site on the surface of the nerve cell.

Ureter: The tube extending from the renal pelvis to the urinary bladder.

Urethra: The tube extending from the urinary bladder to the exterior.

Urethral process: An extension of the urethra beyond the penis as in the stallion and ruminants.

Urinary space: The cavity between the capsular epithelium and the glomerular epithelium of a renal corpuscle.

Urodeum: The portion of the cloaca of a chicken into which urinary wastes are deposited.

Uropygial gland (preen gland): A holocrine gland that produces an oily secretion and is located dorsally within the base of the tail of the chicken.

Uterine gland: A simple, tubular gland within the endometrium of the uterus.

Utriculus: Function same as for sacculus.

Uveal trabecular meshwork: One of three meshworks of connective tissue, within the filtration angle of the eye, whose cavities are filled with aqueous humor.

Vacuolar cell: A cell of the cortex of the chicken ovary containing numerous fat vacuoles and a pyknotic nucleus. Collections of these cells may represent the remnants of a postovulatory follicle.

Vagina (of the chicken oviduct): The segment of the oviduct that opens into the urodeum of the cloaca.

Vane (of a feather): The most prominent feature of a contour feather. It is formed of barbs and interlocking barbules positioned on opposite sides of the rachis.

Vas deferens: The sperm duct that extends from the testis to the urethra.

Vasa vasorum: Blood vessels within the wall of a blood vessel.

Vasa recta: Straight, thin-walled, large diameter blood vessels located within the medulla of the kidney.

Vascular tunic (uvea): The middle layer of the wall of the eye.

Vascular layer (of choroid): The portion of the choroid layer of the eye that contains numerous blood vessels.

Ventral root: The motor portion of a spinal nerve that arises from the ventrolateral part of the spinal cord.

Venule: A small, thin-walled vein.

Vestibular membrane: A thin, epithelial membrane separating the cochlear duct from the scala vestibuli of the inner ear.

Vestibule: An entrance chamber, e.g., of the nose, inner ear, or vulva.

Villus: A finger-shaped process, e.g., intestinal villus.

Visceral pleura: The serous membrane covering the surface of the lung.

Vocal ligament: A band of elastic fibers enclosed in a fold of a mucous membrane.

Volkmann canal: In the diaphysis of a long bone, any transverse channel connecting two haversian canals or piercing the shaft of the bone.

Vulva: The external genitalia of the female mammal; it includes the vestibule, labia, and clitoris.

Wall (of hoof): The part of the hoof that is visible when the digit is on the ground.

Wattle: A fleshy appendage of the skin as in the throat region of the neck of a chicken, goat, or pig.

White line: The junction, at the surface of the ground, of the wall and sole of the horse's hoof.

White matter: The part of the brain or spinal cord containing numerous myelinated neuronal processes.

White pulp: The scattered but numerous concentrations of diffuse and nodular lymphatic tissue found throughout the red pulp of the spleen.

x.s.: Cross section.

Z band (line): The boundary between adjacent sarcomeres of a myofibril; structurally, it represents the point at which the actin filaments of adjacent sarcomeres are in contact with the Z filament.

Zona fasciculata: The thickest portion of the adrenal cortex; located between the zona glomerulosa or zona intermedia and the zona reticularis.

Zona glomerulosa (zona multiformis): The outermost portion of the adrenal cortex.

Zona intermedia: The portion of the adrenal cortex located between the zona glomerulosa and the zona fasciculata.

Zona pellucida: An acidophilic membrane separating an oocyte from the cumulus oophorus.

Zona reticularis: The innermost portion of the adrenal cortex located between the zona fasciculata and the adrenal medulla.

Zonary placenta: A placenta, found in carnivores, that is wrapped around the chorionic sac in the manner of a cummerbund.

Zone of calcification: The portion of the epiphyseal disc where the cartilage matrix becomes infiltrated by calcium salts.

Zone of hypertrophy: The portion of an epiphyseal disc where the chondrocytes become enlarged.

Zone of multiplication (proliferation): The portion of an epiphyseal disc where condrocytes are duplicated.

Zone of ossification: The portion of an epiphyseal disc where cartilage is being replaced by bone.

Zone of reserve cartilage: The portion of an epiphyseal disc that is attached to the bone of the epiphysis.

Zonular fibers: Collagenous suspensory fibers that extend from the capsule of the lens to the ciliary processes.

BIBLIOGRAPHY

Adam, W.S., Calhoun, M.L., Smith, E.M., and Stinson, A.W.: Microscopic Anatomy of the Dog: A Photographic Atlas. Springfield, IL, Charles C. Thomas, 1970.

Amann, R.P., Johnson, L., and Pickett, B.W.: Connection between the seminiferous tubules and the efferent ducts in the stallion. Am. J. Vet. Res., 38:1571, 1977.

Amoroso, E.C.: Histology of the placenta. Br. Med. Bull., 17:81, 1961.

Arey, L.B.: Human Histology. 4th Ed. Philadelphia, W.B. Saunders, 1974.

Banks, W.J.: Applied Veterinary Histology. 2nd Ed. Baltimore, Williams & Wilkins, 1986.

Björkman, N.H.: Fine structure of the fetal-maternal area of exchange in the epitheliochorial and endotheliochorial type of placentation. Acta Anat., 86(Suppl. 1):1, 1973.

Bloom, W., and Fawcett, D.W.: A Textbook of Histology. 10th Ed. Philadelphia, W.B. Saunders, 1975.

Calhoun, M.L.: The microscopic anatomy of the digestive tract of Gallus domesticus. Iowa State Coll. J. Sci., 7:261, 1933.

Cole, H.H., and Cupps, P.T. (eds.): Reproduction in Domestic Animals. Vol. 1. New York, Academic Press, 1959.

Cole, H.H., and Cupps, P.T. (eds.): Reproduction in Domestic Animals. New York, Academic Press, 1969.

Czarnecki, C.M., and Hammer, R.F.: Auto-tutorial Laboratory Guide. Microscopic Anatomy of Domestic Animals. St. Paul, MN, University of Minnesota, 1978.

Dellmann, H., and Brown, E.M.: Textbook of Veterinary Histology. 3rd Ed. Philadelphia, Lea & Febiger, 1993.

Delly, J.G.: Photography Through the Microscope. 7th Ed. Rochester, NY, Eastman Kodak, 1980.

Department of Anatomy: Histology Laboratory Manual (Microscopic Anatomy, VAN. 306). Ames, IA, Iowa State University, 1987.

Di Fiore, M.S.H.: Atlas of Human Histology. 5th Ed. Philadelphia, Lea & Febiger, 1981.

Elias, H.: Comparison of duodenal glands in domestic animals. Am. J. Vet. Res., 8:311, 1947.

Evans, H.E., and Christensen, G.C.: Miller's Anatomy of the Dog. 2nd Ed. Philadelphia, W.B. Saunders, 1979.

Gartner, L.P., and Hiatt, J.L.: Atlas of Histology. Baltimore, Williams & Wilkins, 1987.

Geneser, F.: Color Atlas of Histology. Philadelphia, Lea & Febiger, 1989.

Gentle, M.J.: The lingual taste buds of Gallus Domesticus L. Br. Poult. Sci., 12:245, 1971.

Getty, R.: Sisson and Grossman's The Anatomy of the Domestic Animals. Vol. 1. 5th Ed. Philadelphia, W.B. Saunders, 1975.

Ham, A.W., and Cormack, D.H.: Histology. 8th Ed. Philadelphia, J.B. Lippincott, 1979.

Hammersen, F.: Sabotta/Hammersen. Histology. A Color Atlas of Microscopic Anatomy. 3rd Ed. Baltimore, Urban & Schwarzenberg, 1985.

Hamre, C.J.: Origin and differentiation of heterophil, eosinophil and basophil leukocytes of chickens. Anat. Rec., 112:339, 1952.

Hodges, R.D.: The Histology of the Fowl. New York, Academic Press, 1974.

Huntley, J.F.: Mast cells and basophils: A review of their heterogeniety and function. J. Comp. Path., 107:349, 1992.

Jain, N.C.: Schalm's Veterinary Hematology. 4th Ed. Philadelphia, Lea & Febiger, 1986.

Junqueira, L.C., and Carneiro, J.: Basic Histology. 2nd Ed. Los Altos, CA, Lange Medical Publications, 1980.

Kelly, D.E., Wood, R.L., and Enders, A.C.: Bailey's Textbook of Microscopic Anatomy. 18th Ed. Baltimore, Williams & Wilkins, 1984.

Lawson, D.D., Nixon, G.S., Noble, H.W., and Weipers, W.L.: Dental anatomy and histology of the dog. Res. Vet. Sci., 1:201, 1960.

Leeson, T.S., and Leeson, C.R.: A Brief Atlas of Histology. Philadelphia, W.B. Saunders, 1979.

Lewis, H.B., and Rebar, A.H.: Bone Marrow Evaluation in Veterinary Practice. St. Louis, Ralston Purina, 1979.

Lindenmaier, P., and Kare, M.R.: The taste end-organs of the chicken. Poult. Sci., 38:545, 1959.

Lucas, A.M., and Jamroz, C.: Atlas of Avian Hematology. Washington, DC, United States Department of Agriculture, 1961.

Lucas, A.M., and Stettenheim, P.R.: Avian Anatomy. Integument. Part I. Washington, DC, United States Department of Agriculture, 1972.

Lucas, A.M., and Stettenheim, P.R.: Avian Anatomy. Integument. Part II. Washington, DC, United States Department of Agriculture, 1972.

Melfi, R.C.: Permar's Oral Embryology and Microscopic Anatomy. 7th Ed. Philadelphia, Lea & Febiger, 1982.

Murphy, C.J.: Raptor ophthalmology. Compend. Contin. Educ. Pract. Vet., 9:241, 1987.

Natt, M.P., and Herrick, C.A.: Variation in the shape of the rodlike granules of the chicken heterophil leukocyte and its possible significance. Poult. Sci., 33:828, 1954.

Nickel, R., Schummer, A., and Seiferle, E. (eds.): Anatomy of the Domestic Birds. Translated by W.G. Siller and P.A.L. Wight. New York, Springer-Verlag, 1977.

Olson, P.N., Behrendt, M.D., and Weiss, D.E.: Reproductive problems in the bitch: Finding answers through vaginal cytology. Vet. Med., 82:344, 1987.

Prince, J.H., Diesem, C.D., Eglitis, I., and Ruskell, G.L.: Anatomy and Histology of the Eye and Orbit in Domestic Animals. Springfield, IL, Charles C. Thomas, 1960.

Rebar, A.H.: Handbook of Veterinary Cytology. St. Louis, Ralston Purina, 1980.

Reith, E.J., and Ross, M.H.: Atlas of Descriptive Histology. 3rd Ed. New York, Harper & Row, 1977.

Rich, L.J.: The Morphology of Canine and Feline Blood Cells, Including Equine References. St. Louis, Ralston Purina, 1976.

Ross, M.H., and Romrell, L.J.: Histology. 2nd Ed. Baltimore, Williams & Wilkins, 1989.

Samuel, C.A., Allen, W.R., and Steven, D.H.: Studies on the equine placenta. I. Development of the microcotyledons. J. Reprod. Fertil., 41:441, 1974.

Seely, J.C.: The harderian gland. Lab. Anim., 16:33, 1987.

Shackleford, J.M., and Wilborn, W.H.: Ultrastructure of bovine parotid glands. J. Morphol., 127:453, 1969.

Sloss, M.W.: The microscopic anatomy of the digestive tract of Sus scrofa domestica. Am. J. Vet. Res., 1:578, 1954.

Smith, R.F.: Microscopy and Photomicrography. A Practical Guide. New York, Appleton-Century-Crofts, 1982.

Stedman, T.L.: Illustrated Stedman's Medical Dictionary. 24th Ed. Baltimore, Williams & Wilkins, 1983.

Strickland, J.H., and Calhoun, M.L.: The integumentary system of the cat. Am. J. Vet. Res., *24*:1018, 1963.

Stump, J.E.: Anatomy of the normal equine foot, including microscopic features of the laminar region. J. Am. Vet. Med. Assoc., *151*:1588, 1967.

Sturkie, P.D. (ed.): Avian Physiology. 3rd Ed. New York, Springer-Verlag, 1976.

Trautmann, A., and Fiebiger, J.: Fundamentals of the Histology of Domestic Animals. Translated and revised by R.E. Habel and E.L. Biberstein. Ithaca, NY, Comstock, 1952.

Trautmann, A., and Fiebiger, J.: Fundamentals of the Histology of Domestic Animals. Translated and revised by R.E. Habel and E.L. Biberstein. Ithaca, NY, Comstock, 1957.

Webb, A.J., and Calhoun, M.L.: The microscopic anatomy of the skin of mongrel dogs. Am. J. Vet. Res., *15*:274, 1954.

Weiss, L. : Cell and Tissue Biology, A Textbook of Histology. 6th Ed. Baltimore, Munich, Urban & Schwarzenberg, 1988.

Weiss, L.: The red pulp of the spleen: Structural basis of blood flow. Clin. Haematol., *12*:375, 1983.

Weiss, L., and Greep, R.O.: Histology. 4th Ed. New York, McGraw-Hill, 1977.

Wheater, P.R., Burkitt, H.G., and Daniels, V.G.: Functional Histology. A Text and Colour Atlas. New York, Churchill Livingstone, 1979.

INDEX

Page numbers in *italics* denote figures.

Cartilaginous frame, *267*
Cartilaginous tracheal ring, *186, 187*
Caruncle, 222, *231*
Cat
  blood, *30, 31*
  bone, *22, 23, 24, 25*
  bone marrow, *39–40*
  cardiovascular system, *60, 61, 62, 66*
  connective tissue, *15*
  digestive system, *125, 127, 132, 138, 140, 141, 143, 144, 146, 147, 149, 150, 152*
  endocrine system, *194, 199*
  epithelium, *10, 11*
  eye, *250, 252*
  female reproductive system, *225, 229, 237, 238*
  integument, *88, 92, 94, 102, 103*
  lymphatic system, *72, 73, 83*
  male reproductive system, *214*
  muscle, *44*
  nervous system, *48, 53, 54*
  respiratory system, *180, 182, 183, 184, 185*
  urinary system, *167, 171*
Cationic (basic) stain, 3
Caudal larynx (syrinx), 176, *187, 188*
Caudal region, pars distalis, 193, *200, 201*
Cavernous space
  female reproductive system, *237*
  male reproductive system, 204, *213, 214, 215, 216*
Cavernous vein, *178*
Cavity of air sac, *189*
Cavity of lens, *257*
Cavity of Rathke's pouch, 191, 192, *194, 195*
Cavity of renal pelvis, *169, 170*
Cavity of vitreous humor, 245, *257*
Cecal band, 121, *148*
Cecal tonsil, 83
Cecum, 67, 120, *147, 148, 159*
Cellular tapetum lucidum, 246
Cementum, *123*
Centering slides, 3, 6
Central artery, *79, 80*
Central canal, *49, 50, 54, 55*
Central lacteal, *142, 146*
Central layer, *118*
Central nervous system, 45
Central pallor, *27, 28*
Central vein
  digestive system, *152, 153, 161*
  urinary system, *164*
Centroacinar cell, *155, 156*
Cephalic region, pars distalis, 193, *200*
Cerebellum, *46, 48, 201*
Cerebral cortex, *46*
Cerebrospinal fluid, *47*
Ceruminous gland, *263*
Cervix, 222, *236*
Cheek, *122*
Chestnut, 87, *107*
Chicken
  blood, 28–29, *35–36*
  bone, *24*

bone marrow, 38, *40*
cardiovascular system, 61, *67*
cartilage, *20*
connective tissue, *15*
digestive system, 121, *156–161*
ear, 262, *267*
endocrine system, 193, *200–202*
erythrocyte, average size, 7, 28
eye, *247–248, 257–260*
female reproductive system, 223–224, *239–243*
integument, 87, *112–118*
lymphatic system, 70–71, *83–84*
male reproductive system, 205, *217–219*
nervous system, *54, 55*
respiratory system, 176–177, *185–189*
urinary system, 164–165, *173–174*
Chief cell
  digestive system, 120, *137, 138, 139, 140, 158*
  endocrine system, 192, *198, 202*
Chondrocyte, 19, *20, 66*
Chorioallantoic connective tissue, *233*
Chorioallantoic membrane (CAM), 222, *232, 234, 235*
Chorioallantoic villus, *234, 235, 236*
Choriocapillary layer, 246, *253, 254, 259*
Chorion laeve, *232, 234*
Choroid, 245, 246, *247, 249, 252, 253, 259*
Choroid plexus, *48*
Chromaffin cell, *200*
Chromaffin (medullary) tissue, 193
Chromophil, 191, *200*
Chromophobe, 191, *195, 196, 200*
Cilia
  endocrine system, *198*
  female reproductive system, *228, 231, 236*
  male reproductive system, *218, 219*
  nervous system, *50*
  stereocilia, *210, 262*
Ciliary body, 245, 246, *247, 250, 257, 258*
Ciliary muscle, 246, *249, 250*
Ciliary process, 246, *249, 250, 251, 257*
Ciliated cell, *201, 242*
Ciliated epithelium, *241*
Ciliated pseudostratified columnar epithelium, *10*, 176, 177
Circular muscle, *229*
Circumanal gland, 120, *149, 150, 151*
Circumferential lamellae, 21, *24*
Circumvallate papilla, 119, *126*
Classic lobule, 120
Claw, 87, *106, 117*
Claw fold, *106*
Clear cell, *101*
Clearing specimens, 1, *2*
Clitoris, 223
Cloaca, 121, *160, 164, 165, 205, 240*
Cochlea, *266, 267*
Cochlear canal, *262*
Cochlear duct, 262, *266*
Cochlear nerve, *266, 267*
Collagen, 21
Collagenous band, *104*

capillary, *172*
capsular (parietal) epithelium, 164, *167, 168*
capsule, 163, *166, 167*
cavity of renal pelvis, *169, 170*
central (intralobular) vein, 164
chicken, 164–165, *173–174*
cloaca, 164, 165
collecting duct, *174*
collecting tubule, 163, 164–165, *167, 168, 169, 170, 171, 174*
columnar epithelium, 163
connective tissue, *167*
connective tissue (capsule of), 163
cortex, kidney, 163, *166, 168, 173, 174*
cortical nephrons, 164
distal convoluted cell, 164
distal convoluted tubule, 163, *167, 168, 173, 174*
efferent arteriole, *169*
erythrocyte, *171, 174*
fat vacuole, *167*
glomerular (visceral) epithelium, 164, *167, 174*
glomerulus, 164
Henle's loop, 164, *169, 170, 171, 174*
hilus region, 164
intralobular vein, *173*
juxtaglomerular cell, 164, *168*
kidney, 163–164, *173*
lamina propria, 164, *171, 172*
lobule, 164
loop of Henle, 164, *169, 170, 171, 174*
lymphatic tissue, *174*
macula densa, 164, *167, 168, 169*
mammals, 163–164, *166–172*
medulla, kidney, 163, 164, *166, 169, 170, 171*
medullary cone, 165, *173, 174*
medullary nephrons, 164
medullary tracts, 165
mesangial cell, 164, *174*
mucosa, 164
mucous connective tissue, *171*
mucous gland, *172*
muscularis, 164, *171, 172, 174*
muscularis mucosae, *172*
nephrons, 164
papillary duct, 163, *169, 170, 171*
pars convoluta (cortical labyrinth), 163, *166*
pars radiata, *166, 169*
perilobular collecting duct, 165
proximal convoluted tubule, 163, 164, *167, 168, 169, 173, 174*
pseudostratified epithelium, 163, 165, *174*
renal corpuscle, 164, *166, 167, 173*
renal papilla, 163, *169, 170*
renal pelvis, 163
reticular fiber, *171*
serosa, *174*
smooth muscle, *167*
subcapsular vein, *167*
submucosa, 164, *172*
superficial cortex, *167*
transitional epithelium, *171, 172*
urachus, *171*

ureter, 164, 165, *171, 172, 174*
urethra, 163, 164
urinary bladder, 164, *172*
urinary space, 164, *167, 168, 169, 174*
urodeum, 164
vasa recta, 164, *169, 170, 171*
Urodeum, *160*, 164
Uropygial (preen) gland, 87, *117, 118*
Uterine (endometrial) gland, 222, *234, 235*
Uterine gland, *59*
Uterine horn, *229, 230, 231*
Uterus, 222, *231, 234, 240, 243*
Utriculus, 262
Uvea (vascular tunic), 245
Uveal meshwork (pectinate ligament), 246, 247, *250, 251, 254, 257, 258*
Uveal trabecular meshwork, 246, *251*

Vacuolar cell, 223, *239*
Vacuolated cell, *100*
Vacuole, 29, *35, 243*
Vagina, 222–223, 224, *237, 240, 243*
Vaginal smear, *238, 239*
Valves, 58, *60, 62, 65, 67*
Vane, 87
Vas deferens (ductus deferens), 204, 205, *210, 211, 219*
Vasa recta, 164, *169, 170, 171*
Vasa vasorum, 57, *64*
Vascular layer, choroid, 246, *250, 253, 254*
Vascular sinusoid, 37, 38
Vascular stratum (stratum cavernosum), 204, *212*
Vascular tunic (uvea), 245
Vein
    bone, *25*
    cardiovascular system, 57, 59, 60, 61, *62, 67*
    cavernous vein, *178*
    central vein, digestive system, *152, 153, 161*
    central vein, urinary system, 164
    digestive system, *136, 148, 152, 153, 161*
    female reproductive system, *230*
    intralobular vein, *173*
    medium vein, 57, *61, 62*
    portal vein, *62, 152, 153*
    pulmonary vein, *185*
    respiratory system, *178, 185*
    small vein, 57, *59, 60*
    subcapsular vein, *167*
    urinary system, 164, *167, 173*
Vena cava, *64*
Venous sinus, 70, 79
Ventral boundary of third ventricle (median eminence), 192, 193, *194*
Ventral plate, *117*
Ventral root, *55*
Ventriculus (gizzard), 121, *158*
Venule
    cardiovascular system, 57, 59, 60, *67*
    integument, *98*
    lymphatic system, 70, *77*
    muscle, *42*
    nervous system, *48*
    postcapillary venule, 70, *77*

Verniers, for relocating structures, 6
Vesicles, *84*
Vestibular epithelium, *185, 237*
Vestibular fold, *73*
Vestibular gland, *237*
Vestibular (Reissner's) membrane, *262, 266*
Vestibule
    ear, 262, *264*
    female reproductive system, 223, *238*
    respiratory system, *175, 176*
Vestigial cavity, 192
Villus
    chorioallantoic villus, *234, 235, 236*
    digestive system, 120, 121, *141, 143, 144, 146, 147, 159,*
       160
    female reproductive system, *234, 235, 236*
    lymphatic system, *72, 73, 83*
    male reproductive system, *210*
    nervous system, *48*
Villous surfaces, 222
Visceral (glomerular) epithelium, 164, *167, 174*
Visceral pleura, 176, *184*
Visceral prepuce, *217*
Vocal fold, *180*
Vocal ligament, *180*
Volkmann's canal, *24, 25*
Vulva, 223

Wall of hoof, *106, 110*
Waterbath, straightening sections on, 1, 2, 3
Wattle, 87, *114*
Weigert stain (resorcin fuchsin), 3
White blood cell. *See* Leukocyte
White line, hoof, 108, *109*
White matter, *46, 49, 54, 55*
White pulp, 70–71, *79, 81, 83*
Wright stain (Romanovsky), 3

Yolk sphere, *240*

Z band, 41, *43*
Zona fasciculata, 192, *199, 200*
Zona glomerulosa (zone multiformis), 192, *199, 200*
Zona intermedia, 192, *199, 200*
Zona pellucida, 221, *225, 226*
Zona reticularis, 192, *199, 200*
Zonary placenta, 222, *232, 233, 234*
Zone multiformis (zona glomerulosa), 192, *199, 200*
Zone of calcification, 23, *24*
Zone of hypertrophy, 23, *24*
Zone of multiplication, 23, *24*
Zone of ossification, 23, *24*
Zone of reserve cartilage, *23*
Zonular fiber, 245, 246, *249, 251, 257, 258*